Eating
SIMPLY

EATING SIMPLY

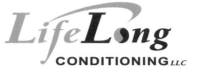

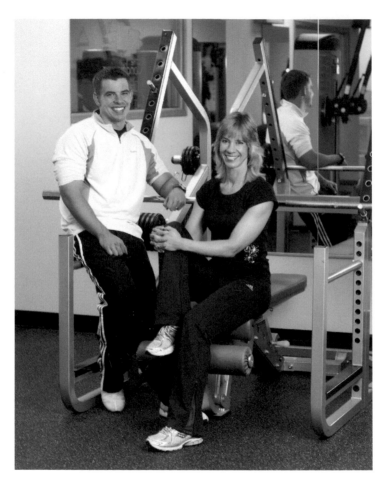

Credits

Concept and Design by Dianne Bailey, CSCS and Grant Pettegrew, CSCS.

Photographs pages 2, 83, 84, 86, 89-92 © 2013 Barry Staver

Photographs on pages 55, 58, 59, 60 © 2013 Larry DiPasquale

Photographs on front and back cover and pages 4, 6, 8, 12, 14, 19, 20, 25, 26, 34, 44-47, 49, 50, 58, 61, 63, 65, 66, 71, 76, 78, 80 © 2013 James Bailey

TABLE OF CONTENTS

PREFACE ● ● ● ● ● ● ● ● ● ● ● ● ● ● ● ● ● ●

Let's start by agreeing on some simple ideas:

Eating should be pleasurable.

Eating should be flavorful.

Eating should provide nutrition to your body.

Eating should not take excessive amounts of your time.

Eating should support your goals.

Eating should not be stressful.

Eating should be simple.

Healthy eating, however, has unfortunately been associated with "complicated, time consuming, tasteless and boring." This doesn't need to be the case. You can eat well and enjoy it, believe me! This book is meant to rescue all the refugees who have run away from healthy eating and are stuck in the mire of fast food purgatory. You know that you can change your body and be healthier . . . if only the food thing didn't have to happen. You want to feel better, look better, maybe drop a few pounds and enjoy being active . . . but each time you try, the food part trips you up. Maybe you think you are too busy to fix your own food. Maybe you feel overwhelmed and uncomfortable in the kitchen. Maybe you've just gotten lazy. This book is for you. It is meant to be a simple guide, a compass that points you in the direction of better health. It is not a detailed map or GPS unit that tells you specifically the turns you must make in exactly the right order. This book will not dive into the scientific specifics of nutrition. This book is designed to be simple. So you actually have some responsibility in this journey to decide which roads you want to explore and travel. Together, we'll discover that eating simply can become the basis for a happier, healthier, spicier you!

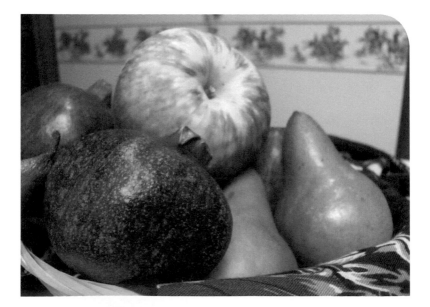

CHAPTER 1

EATING SIMPLY . . . IS SIMPLY EATING

Can you break away from the shackles of fast, convenient and unhealthy? Fast and convenient sound good, don't they? But do you ever stop to think about "unhealthy?" What are you really doing to your body when you eat commercially prepared "food?"

Eating Simply does not come from a box.

The food industry has tried to box us up for years. I'm trying to open your mind and help you see what's real. Since the 1960's, we have tried to make things in the kitchen as fast and easy as possible. We created TV dinners, added trans-fat to all kinds of boxed food so that it would be "shelf-stable", added salt to preserve and sugar to make things edible. We worked really hard to become as pre-processed as possible so all of the work was done before we ever stepped foot into the kitchen. This may seem like it made eating simple for everyone. And on one level, it did. But on a deeper level, this kind of simplification created a maelstrom of problems for every cell in our bodies. You see, the processing actually created non-food instead of simple food. You might as well sit down and eat a bowl of sawdust . . . it would certainly be simple to prepare and would provide just as much nutrition for your body as the packaged, processed, simple food that you can purchase. You've heard of "empty calories," right? And I'm sure you associated that phrase with sugar-laden desserts and/ or alcohol. You need to start associating that phrase with pre-packaged foods as well. It may feel like you are eating a meal; you may feel full and even satisfied when you are done; there may have even been some vegetables involved . . . but your body did not recognize what you ate as nutrition for its essential processes. In the extreme, your body may have even considered some of what you ate as an invader to be attacked. I know that sounds weird and overly suspicious. An inflammatory response may result because what you've eaten is not recognized as "food", but rather as a foreign substance that needs to be isolated and removed before it causes further damage to our cells.

Supporting real health by eating real food does not need to be intimidating.

Yes, you actually have to take some time and effort to plan and prepare, but you don't have to continually consider "what is in this piece of broccoli?" Or, "what has been removed from this piece of broccoli?" I will briefly mention that I believe you should move towards organic products as much as you can so you are not ingesting unnecessary added chemicals. Right now, however, commit to changing from pre-processed easy to natural, real eating . . . simply.

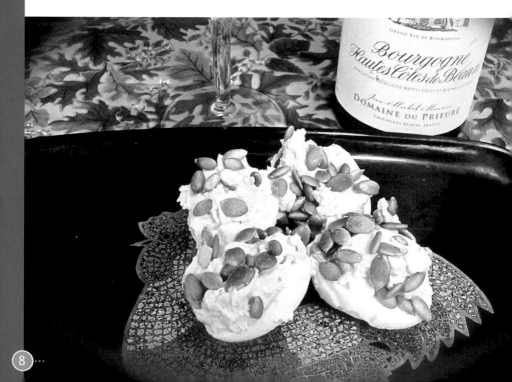

EATING SIMPLY IS NOT EATING OUT

In the old days, "Fast Food" meant that the deer you were hunting kept getting away from you! No, seriously, the whole concept of fast food boggles my mind. I watch people sitting in their cars, waiting to order what they think will feed their bodies and I wonder if they realize that it's all a mirage. Damaging fats, mountains of sodium and rivers of high fructose corn syrup come through the fast food window . . . but not anything that will actually feed your body. Remember that a restaurant's goal is not to keep you healthy. Their goal is to make money. And they do that by creating "food" that tastes good and makes you want to have more. More than you need, actually. There is a song performed by Kathy Mattea* with the lyrics, "Standing knee-deep in a river and dying of thirst." That's exactly what is happening to you when you rely on fast food to feed your body. No real nutrition is reaching your cells. You are drowning your body with un-necessary and harmful ingredients and yet your body ends up malnourished. Each time you take your kids through the "drive-thru" for a meal because you just don't have the time to prepare real food, you are dumping garbage into their systems that takes months to exit their bodies. Some "treat", huh? On the other hand, with just a little planning and preparation, your family can eat real food on the way to the soccer game. By making our Chicken Orzo Salad (recipe on pg. 61) on the weekend and storing it in the refrigerator in individual sized food containers, all you have to do is grab the containers and some forks and throw them into a cooler with some ice. Throw in some oranges for dessert and you have a healthy, fast, easy dinner that will feed your bodies instead of causing more damage. And I bet it will even be less expensive!

Does fast food make you feel fast? Or sluggish? It is possible to eat simply just as fast . . . with the added benefit of speeding up your metabolism! Now that's speed we can all appreciate.

---

* Knee Deep in a River (Dying of Thirst) by Bob McDill, Dickey Lee and Bucky I Jones. Performed by Kathy Mattea on "Lonesome Standard Time"® 1992, Mercury Records, a Division of UMG Recordings, Inc.

EATING SIMPLY DOESN'T COUNT . . . CALORIES, THAT IS!

What you eat is more important than the calorie count. Let's say you need 1500 calories each day to survive. Would your body function at its best if you ate 1500 calories of donuts? Or drank 1500 calories of vodka? No! You know that's silly. And yet, people still fixate on that caloric balance equation: if you want to lose weight, you have to consume fewer calories than you expend. That view is myopic. You must feed your body the nutrients it needs to think, to move, to encourage it to utilize any "excess body fat" as fuel so you can become leaner and stronger.

I want you to learn to eat with an attitude towards "yes" and not continue to approach food with the idea of "can't." Eating simply does, in fact, encourage eating lots of different foods. You should include all of the macronutrients in every meal: a lean protein, a complex carbohydrate and a quality fat. I will give you some lists to choose from so you can build your own meals with this idea in mind (see pg. 42). The lean protein is important so that your body can continually repair, re-build and replace. The complex carbohydrate is necessary to give you energy to complete all of your tasks each day . . . especially your mental tasks! The quality fat helps your body regulate hormone, enzyme, and mineral activity so all your "systems" stay strong. You see, eating is all about feeding your body the fuel that it needs to function. So, start thinking in terms of how to build the best meals every day.

Eating simply actually makes your day simpler and less stressful because you don't have to bother with counting calories. The only things you need to count are the number of meals you are eating each day. Ideally, you should be eating every 3 to 3 ½ hours, which works out to five or six small meals. If each meal contains a lean protein, a complex carbohydrate and a quality fat, you are doing more good for your body than you ever would by restricting calories.

EATING SIMPLY IS SIMPLY EATING . . .

And taking back control of your life!

I hope by now you are starting to understand that the food manufacturers, the food vendors and the government are not really all that concerned about your health. (Oh, that sounds like a great conspiracy theory!) The bottom line is this: You have to start taking responsibility for the food you consume. If you continue to abdicate that responsibility and consume pre-packaged, pre-assembled, and pre-cooked - basically pre-digested meals - then your body will break down faster, you will continue to struggle with illness, weight and energy issues, and you won't live the life you were meant to live. Heavy stuff, huh? But we really are talking about basic, cellular health. Garbage In . . . Garbage Out. What you eat really is this important. Of course, I want my clients to exercise (see the Afterward, Exercising Simply). Movement is critical. But real transformation occurs when you take control of both of these things: what you eat and how you move.

The rest of this book is designed to help you take your first steps towards simply eating. It's not complicated. You won't find lengthy discussions of specific ingredients to incorporate into your diet or to avoid. You will find some simple ideas for organizing your "food life" and some simple recipes to try. I want this book to be a cornerstone for your daily life so you can start to take control of the food you are regularly putting into your body. This is not hard-core nutritional science, but rather an overall lifetime structure for eating that should be fleshed out in the way that suits you and your life the best. So relax. Soon you will be creating fun, tasty meals that are simple to fix.

REMEMBER · · · · ·

- Eating should be pleasurable.
- Eating should be flavorful.
- Eating should provide nutrition to your body.
- Eating should not take excessive amounts of your time.
- Eating should support your goals.
- Eating should not be stressful.
- Eating should be simple.

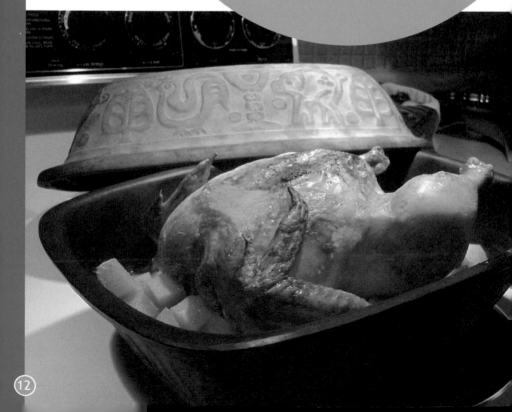

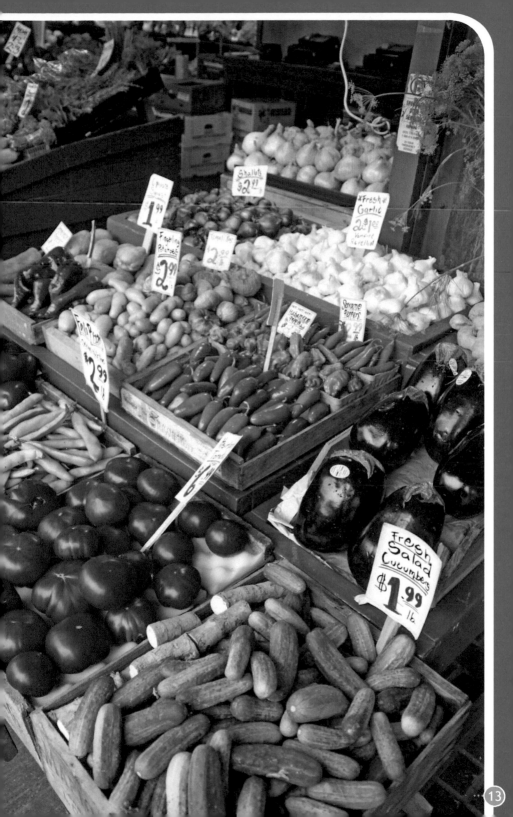

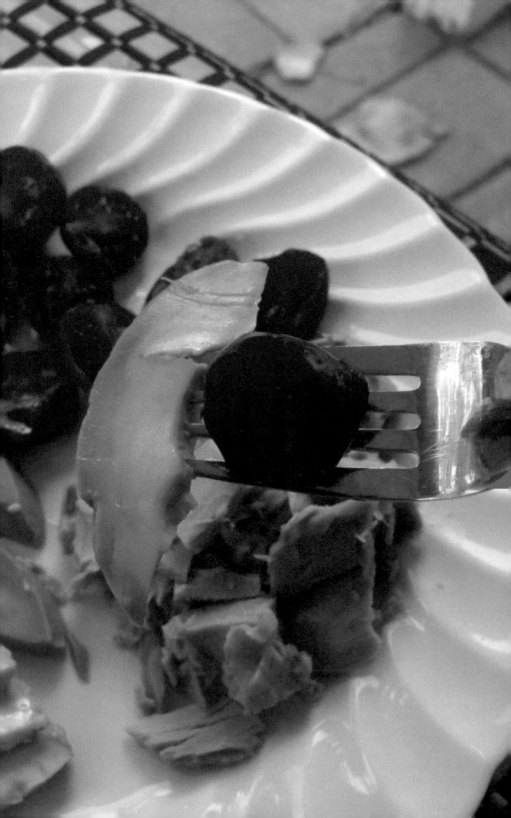

CHAPTER 2

THE FIVE TENETS OF EATING SIMPLY

Seriously, I wanted to say the "5 Commandments of Eating Simply." That sounds just a little too Biblical, doesn't it? But the importance of these 5 tenets is tremendous. When you understand these and start to implement them into your every day life, you will start to feel fully alive.

---

1. EAT FREQUENTLY

You need to be fueling your body every 3 to 3 ½ hours. This may not sound "simple," but by doing this, you are reassuring your body that it does NOT need to store fat because it will get fed regularly. If you restrict food, your body begins to believe there is a famine and you can't find enough food to feed it. So, in order to survive, the body responds by cooling down its metabolic fires. One of the results of this slow-down is the preference for storing fuel because after all, you don't know where your next meal is coming from! So instead of the intended consequence of not eating as much – losing fat – you are actually encouraging your body to store the food it does get as fat. Of course, when you eat frequently, it doesn't mean you gorge yourself every few hours. The portions you choose should be just enough that you are indeed hungry again in 3 hours. It takes a little time to figure what it is enough for you, but this is where you really need to listen to your body. Your activity level will dictate your portion needs. If you work at a desk job, you will need less than someone who has a physically demanding job. Remember that your food intake needs to support your goals and your lifestyle. After some trial and error, eating frequently with the right portion size really does become simple . . . if you are willing to take some time planning your meals for the day.

2. EAT NATURALLY

The food you consume should be as natural and unprocessed as possible. Processed food is basically "pre-digested" and does your body more harm than good. Many of the nutrients are destroyed or removed in the process of making food more shelf-stable and/ or attractive for purchase. For example, white flour is easier to use and creates fantastic tasting breads, cakes and cookies. But white flour is made by stripping the hull and the germ off the wheat. Most of the fiber and nutrients of wheat are in the hull and the germ. So you are left with a great tasting, but nutritionally void product. That's why white flour is "enriched." They have to add back some nutritional value!

Your body actually wants to be in charge of the "processing" of the food you give it. When you eat food that comes from a box, the work of processing has already been done, so the food enters your system quickly and causes your blood sugar to rise too quickly. This causes your body to over-react to take care of the excess blood sugar. By eating more naturally and not relying on pre-processed foods, you allow your body to do the work of digesting the way it was intended. The fiber in a whole piece of fruit takes work to process in your gut and it helps mitigate the response to the influx of fructose. A piece of chicken takes much more work to digest than a protein bar. I know this sounds more complicated than simple. Again, it just takes a little planning to make it happen. When you are grilling chicken breast on Saturday for dinner, cook 2 or 3 extra pieces. Then on Monday, grab an orange, a chicken breast and some cucumber slices. Eat half of each of these at "lunch" and eat the other half mid-afternoon. Voila! You are eating frequently and naturally!

3. EAT COMPLETELY

Each "meal" that you eat should be complete and should contain a lean protein, a complex carbohydrate and a good fat. This ensures that each meal is a "thermic" event. In other words, because you are eating as naturally as possible (see #2), your body will have to work hard to digest the food you are eating. It will take time for your body to break the food into the components it can use and then supply the right tissues with the right fuel. This is good! And because each meal contains all the components it needs (and not too much!), your body recognizes that this eating event is a refueling event, so it works to utilize the fuel and not store it. So let's look at the separate pieces that create the whole meal. Lean proteins include chicken, eggs, turkey, fish, buffalo and lean beef. Complex carbohydrates can be broken down into two categories: fibrous carbs and starchy carbs. Fibrous carbs are vegetables. Starchy carbs are whole grains, potatoes and beans. Good fats include olive oil, avocados and nuts. Take a look at our "pick and choose" list (pg.42) to create great, simple meals every time!

4. EAT LESS SUGAR

Okay. For the most part, eating simply is about encouraging you to eat and to eat well. It's not based on "thou shalt nots" and other restrictions. However, I do need to mention the place that sugar has in your life. Read this again. I am not saying "Don't ever eat sugar." In fact, I even included a chapter entitled, "Simply Sweet." So let's talk a little about that addictive white substance called sugar. First of all, it is addictive. The more you eat, the more you crave it. And then it takes more of it to satisfy you. The single bit of chocolate becomes ½ the candy bar and then the whole candy bar and so on. But why do we care? Remember #2 and #3 – eat naturally and completely? Sugar is very processed and extremely easy for your body to dump into the blood stream. Almost no work is needed, and your blood sugar begins to skyrocket immediately! Not only that, if you fill up on sugar calories, you are less likely to eat the things you really need, i.e. lean protein, complex carbs and fats. You begin to cheat your body and it doesn't get the nutrients it needs to be lean and healthy. Sugar also encourages your body to store fat by dramatically increasing blood sugar, which signals insulin, which works really hard to shuttle that sugar into the cells that need it and store the excess for later. Stored energy is also known as fat. So how can you manage your sugar intake simply? Start by learning where sugar is in your diet. You'll be surprised that it is not just in your cookies and donuts. It is also in your bread, your cereal, your ketchup and barbecue sauce. You'll also find large amounts in that "healthy" yogurt you've been eating. And don't forget the beverages you drink every day. Sodas, juices, bottled teas, coffee drinks all have loads of sugar. And one final note that you need to consider . . . fruit has a lot of sugar, too. I know, fruit is natural. And I do want you to enjoy fruit when it is fresh and in season for the vitamins, minerals and fiber that it can provide. You just need to be aware that fruit is really nature's dessert. When you eat it as part of a meal, you can eat an appropriate portion and your body has to work at digesting the complete meal, so the sugar doesn't have a chance to spike your blood sugar. And think about it, how much easier is it to add a slice of watermelon to your plate than to bake a whole cake, frosting and all? So eat simply . . . with just a little sugar on top.

5. EAT TO BE STABLE

This is the compilation of all of the above. By eating small portions of lean protein, complex carbohydrates and quality fats every 3 to 3 ½ hours with minimal sugar intake, you will be stabilizing your blood sugar and not allowing it to go on a roller coaster ride. The food you eat and the portions you allow yourself and the timing in which your meals occur directly affects the hormone production in your body. This hormone regulation is essential to utilizing the food properly for energy and for storing the excess for future use. Stabilizing your blood sugar . . . or making it move in gently undulating patterns is desirable if you want to master your metabolism. Following the tenets of Eating Simply makes this possible.

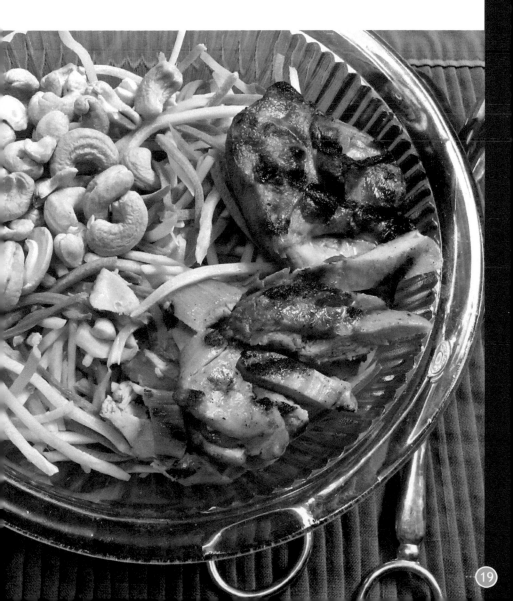

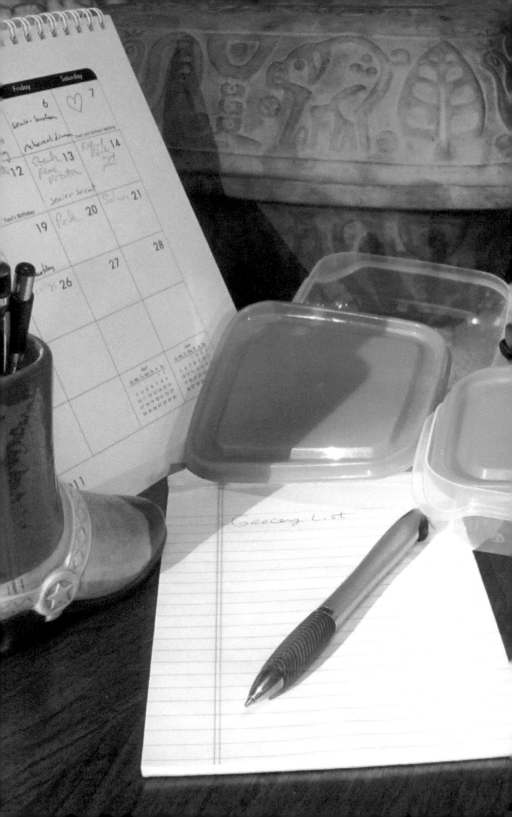

CHAPTER 3

SIMPLY PLANNING

This step cannot be ignored if you want to start implementing
Eating Simply into your life. It may sound cumbersome at first,
but it actually will be very "freeing" when you put the right pieces
in place.

EATING SIMPLY TAKES PLANNING

Real, quality, good-for-you food is not difficult to prepare. But it
does not miraculously appear on your table or in your lunch box,
either. A weekly trip to the grocery store is absolutely necessary.
Having certain "go to" foods available in your pantry is extremely
helpful. Utilizing re-usable containers is essential. Hold on . . . I
can feel your blood pressure rising. The planning process may be
foreign at first, but it becomes second nature quickly. You don't
have to have every meal of every day perfectly planned out. But
you do have to have the right ingredients available so that each
meal you put together can contain the proper macro-nutrients.
Leftovers are a great source of meals throughout each week. If
you are fixing chicken on the grill, just cook 2 or 3 extra pieces.
It doesn't take any extra time to cook them! And then you have
a great lean protein available to include in sandwiches or salads.
Easy, huh? Remember, you are choosing to take control of your
food, instead of your food controlling you. This will not be the last
time you hear me stressing the importance of planning ahead.

SIMPLE EQUIPMENT

Eating simply, like anything else, is easier with the right equipment. Let's talk about food preparation equipment first.

A crockpot is invaluable when you want to create home-cooked meals while you are actually away from home. There are many great cookbooks available that focus on this easy to use cooking device. It takes a little bit of time in the morning to prepare, and then you let it cook all day while you are at work. When you get home, dinner is served! Simple and healthy! I will use my crockpot to cook lean beef for things like fajitas or taco salad. I will also make my own applesauce in the fall with my crockpot. Just peel and slice your apples and fill your crockpot. Let it cook overnight. In the morning, you will wake up to the wonderful smell of apples and easy, healthy applesauce to add to your breakfast.

Chicken can be cooked in the crockpot, too. But it can overcook pretty easily. Another cooking device that is easy to use and helps with healthy dinners is a clay pot. You have to have some time, but clay pot chicken is the easiest, most flavorful way to prepare a whole chicken. Again, there are cookbooks dedicated to this kitchen tool, but all you really have to do is cut up some carrots and onions and add them to the pot. Place the whole chicken on top. Add about ¼ cup of chicken broth. About an hour later, you will have the most flavorful, moist chicken you have ever tasted! Cooking the whole chicken on the weekend when you have extra time provides cooked chicken for lunches throughout the week.

The other equipment that you need for eating simply is a number of differing sizes of food containers and a way to carry those containers with you throughout the day. You can buy Tupperware or Rubbermaid or any other brand of container. You will need some kind of cooling device . . . ice or re-usable freezing units. You will need a cooler or a lunch bag that will keep your containers and freezing units as needed.

If you have these things available, you will be more likely to bring your own food each day to work instead of stopping for "fast food." You will be able to control the amount of sodium, fat and simple carbohydrates you ingest each day. You will be able to increase the amount of vegetables you eat and reduce the reliance on "empty calories" to satisfy your body.

FOOD EXERCISE #1

Plan the entire week and compare at the end.

This is similar to a food journal except that you plan your meals ahead of time instead of just recording as you go. Planning each meal for the week ahead will provide you with a ready-made grocery list and make your trip to the store much more efficient. The time spent planning ahead will actually save you time during the week because you won't be faced with the dreaded question, "What's for dinner?" It will also prevent wasting food because there is a meal for each vegetable and each piece of meat you bought. I bet you have a calendar somewhere in your house. Start planning your meals on that calendar.

Since life always gets in the way, you may only follow it for 5 or 6 days, or whatever may happen. The challenge is to achieve the "perfect week." A week where you create a plan for every meal in the week and you stick to it.

You may find that it will really simplify your life!

Eating Simply Pantry/Refrigerator/Freezer Basics
(Have these things on hand at all times to be able to create meals on a moment's notice.)

OLIVE OIL
BOXED/CANNED BEANS
BOXED/CANNED TOMATOES
SPICES
EGGS
BROWN RICE
OATS
CANNED TUNA
NUTS
LETTUCE
PEANUT BUTTER
ALL-FRUIT JELLY
LOW-SODIUM CHICKEN OR VEGETABLE BROTH
COTTAGE CHEESE
PLAIN YOGURT
FRESH/FROZEN FRUIT
CHICKEN BREASTS
GROUND BEEF
BUTTER
WHOLE WHEAT OR SPELT ENGLISH MUFFINS
WHOLE WHEAT TORTILLAS
MUSTARD
LEMON JUICE
OAT BRAN
FRESH/FROZEN VEGETABLES
MILK
SOY/HOISIN/BBQ SAUCE

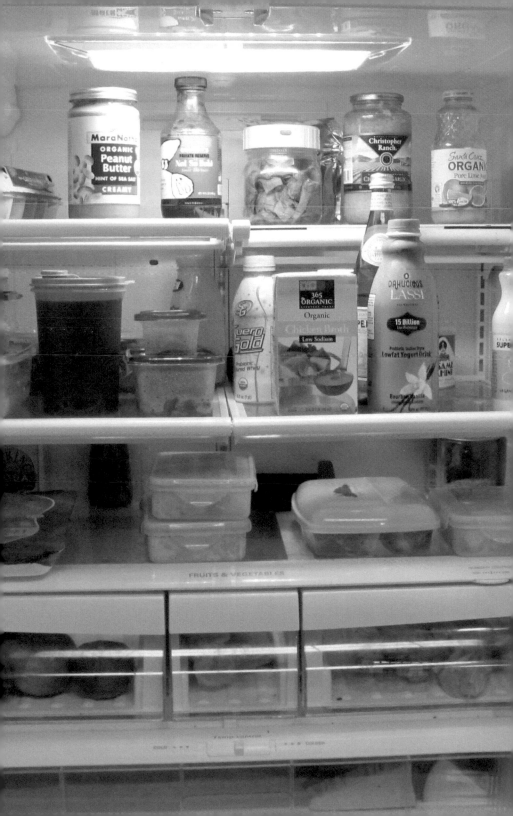

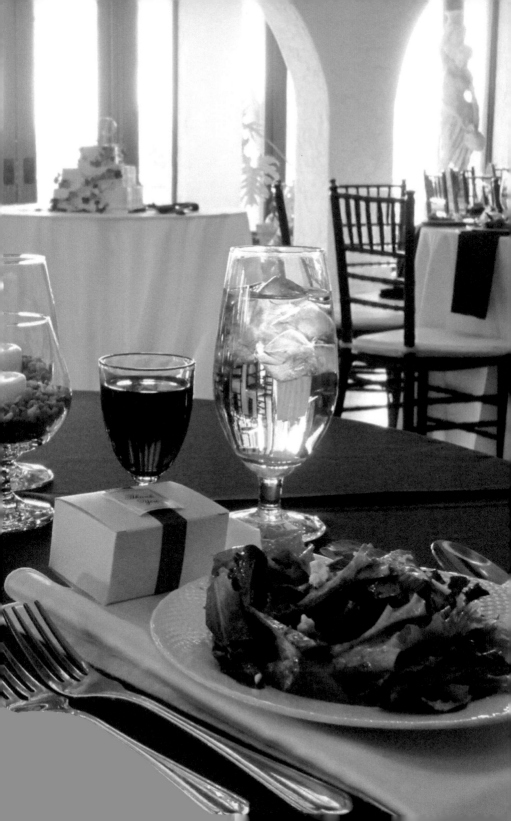

CHAPTER 4

EATING SIMPLY FOR WEIGHT LOSS

Eating Simply is for everyone . . . to feel their best and to look their best. Some of us are on a mission to lose some weight so we can feel and look our best. If you embrace these 4 simple concepts of Eating Simply for weight loss, you will be well on your way to being the best you can be!

If weight (and fat) loss is your main goal, then follow this easy to use "4 corner" checklist when eating. Simply check these off in your mind before you make or order (if you absolutely have to eat out) your meal.

The following tips are simple, yet effective.

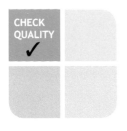 Your first check mark may be the most difficult, yet is certainly the most important. Ensure you are eating lean protein (ideally from an organic source) instead of overly fatty proteins; complex carbohydrates over simple carbohydrates; and good fats over bad fats.

For example, here is a meal that could easily be improved on overall quality:

80/20 Ground beef hamburger patty, white bread bun, cheddar cheese, condiments. Side of potato chips.

Notice the fatty protein (80/20 beef), simple carbs (white bread, potato chips), and bad fats (cheese and chips)

That same meal could look like this instead:

93/7 Organic ground beef or buffalo, whole-wheat bun (possibly a thin one), avocado, condiments. Side of grapes.

This is essentially the same meal, yet made with lean protein (93/7 beef), complex carbs (whole wheat, grapes) and good fats (avocado). You see, you don't have to give up your favorite meals. Just tweak them a bit, and you are helping your body by providing it with the fuel it can use.

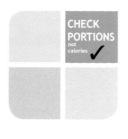

The next step is to check how much you're eating. Even if you are eating quality food, if you eat too much you will gain weight. Eat the burger mentioned before, but with 2 patties, a whole avocado, and a full bowl of grapes and it isn't going to be quite as effective for weight loss.

However, you don't need to count calories! When you are eating frequently, you only need to eat a small portion, because you will fuel your body again in a few hours.

Using the burger example again, you can decrease your portion by using a thin whole-wheat bun, or by using lettuce as a wrap instead. You still consume a delicious burger with a sweet side of grapes, but your overall portion is decreased, helping you achieve your weight and fat loss goal.

When you eat only a couple meals a day, a normal person will experience a wide range on the Eating Simply Hunger Scale, which goes from "Cranky Starving" (0) to "Thanksgiving Stuffed Full" (10).

With only a couple large meals you can easily go from 0-10. However, if you eat simply and frequently, you may only go from 3-7. I can tell you from experience, that this is much more enjoyable.

So a good marker for portion control (if you are eating slowly) is about a 7. Listen to what your body is telling you and don't be afraid to stop eating!

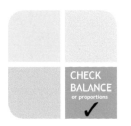

CHECK
BALANCE
or proportions
✓

Before you begin eating, the next checklist item is to look at your plate and check your proportions.

Is your meal balanced?

Is your meal primarily dominated by proteins and fibrous carbohydrates (aka vegetables)?

Are your starchy carbohydrates under 1/3 of your meal?

Every meal may not be perfect, but it is important to check your proportions and ensure they do not consistently get "out of whack."

Having too many simple carbohydrates can spike your blood sugar, creating an eventual crash and thus defeating the purpose of food: To give you energy and support your body!

The macronutrient "balance" of your meal will not only help determine the success of your weight loss goal, but it will also affect how you feel immediately afterwards. And I don't know about you, but I want to feel good after I eat!

• • • **TIP**
Eat slowly so your body can recognize the food and send the satiation signals to your brain.

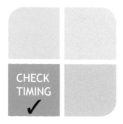

CHECK
TIMING
✓

Your final checklist item is a simple check of the clock. If more than a few hours have passed by, you need to get some food!

Ask yourself these questions:

"Am I eating frequently?"

"Was my last meal 3-4 hours ago?"

"Have I planned ahead and stuck to my schedule?"

These are simple questions to ensure your body is constantly and consistently receiving the fuel it needs to operate. And when I say operate, I am referring not only to the most basic biological functions needed for daily living/survival, but the other functions you want to support for weight and fat loss. Your body needs fuel to recover from exercise, to build metabolism-boosting muscle, and even to burn fat!

Ideally you are eating 4-6 small meals every 3-4 hours, so check the clock and plan your meals ahead of time! If you wake up and eat breakfast at 7am, then your following meals should be at 10am, 1pm, 4pm, and dinner at 7pm. It really is quite simple!

So using the burger example from the "Check Quality" section as an example, let's go through the 4 part checklist to confirm the meal you are about to eat is simple and supporting your goals!

QUALITY

Ideally you choose lean (93/7) ground beef or buffalo, whole wheat bun (thin or not), good vegetables and condiments, and grapes as a side.

PORTION

The patty is reasonably sized (deck of cards or slightly larger) and the bun can be thin or completely eliminated. The grapes are chosen ahead of time so you don't continually "graze".

BALANCE

The protein and vegetables are the largest portion of the meal, with the grapes and bun being the smaller "sides".

TIMING

The last meal consumed was 3 ½ hours earlier, so it is perfect timing!

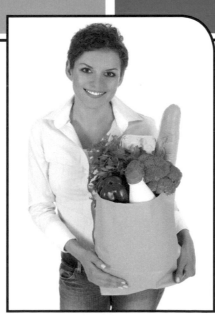

FOOD EXERCISE #2

FOOD JOURNAL FOR 7 DAYS:
Classify as good, bad, and ugly

You are probably familiar with food journaling and the benefits associated with it:

1. It keeps you accountable
2. It opens your eyes to exactly what you are eating each day
3. You are able to see how often you are eating and how long you go without quality sources of the macronutrients (fat, carbs, protein)
4. You are able to compare days of the week and determine where you often fall short (for most people it's the weekend)

In this exercise, you will still be journaling your food, but at the end of the week, you are going to add a little "twist."

After completing 7 full days, review each day through the eyes of Eating Simply and give yourself one of three grades: Good, Bad, or Ugly.

Review quality of food, quantity, proportion, and timing (i.e. the four corners). Don't forget your water too!

Give yourself an honest grade for each day. Make a mental note (or physical if you're that type of person) on how you can improve and then file them into their respective categories.

Ideally you would have a pile of 7 Good days, but we know that isn't realistic. This is a work in progress. But realistically, you would have a few Good, a few Bad, and maybe one Ugly day.

The idea is to continually improve your ratio, resulting in a majority (5-6) Good days, with only a couple (1-2) Bad days and no Ugly days at all.

Do this frequently to track your progress throughout the year. But don't be afraid to give yourself an occasional break so you don't burn out on journaling. Remember, you want eating to be simple and fun, not a constant chore.

SUN MON **TUES** WED **THUR** FRI **SAT!!!**

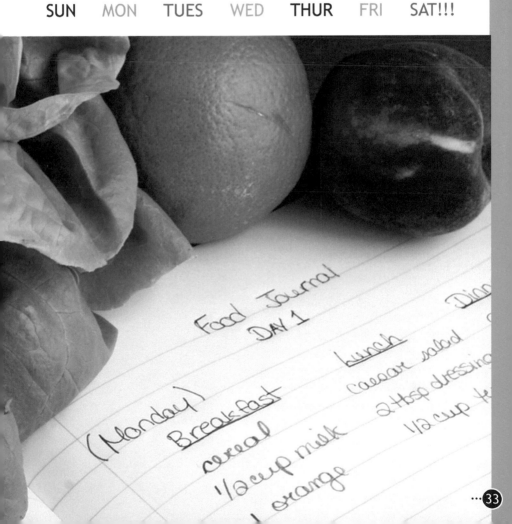

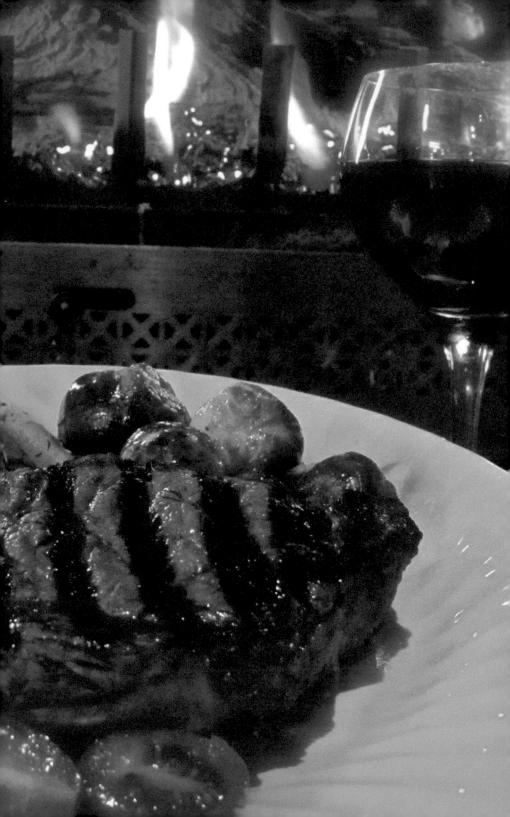

CHAPTER 5

SIMPLY WEEKENDS

Most of us have two nutritional lives: Weekday nutrition and Weekend nutrition. The difference is obvious, but the truth is that people significantly change how and what they eat Saturday-Sunday compared to Monday-Friday.

Weekends vs. Weekdays

The weekdays are subject to routine and convenience. Family schedules are mostly cyclical throughout the week, creating normal and predictable possibilities for dinner. Lunches are usually at the same time, with the same people, whether you work in an office or you stay at home. Adjust the routines to allow for simple eating principles and success will follow.

However, on the weekends, your life changes. Weekends are a random mix of social activities, chores, kid's events, house/yard work, errands, etc. Schedules are constantly crazy and unpredictable, creating havoc instead of routine. And if you are eating well all week long, isn't it frustrating to have the weekend ruin everything you have been working for?

So to avoid a dangerous weekend slide of eating poorly follow these tips:

1. Announce your intentions
Tell your family, friends, or whoever you will be spending the weekend with that you are planning on eating simply, so they are not surprised when you ask to stop at a local restaurant for a quality meal. Let them know where you would like to eat ahead of time, whether it is at a restaurant or at home.

2. Plan ahead

Duh! The more you plan ahead, the better. I told you that it wasn't going to be the last time you would hear this. This is especially essential on the weekends. If you don't know what you are going to eat, you are subject to the will of the day, and thus to the desires of those around you.

3. Choose at least one fun meal

The weekends are about escaping normal routine, having fun and enjoying your friends and family. So choose at least one meal that is out of the ordinary, creating something unique and new to you. Have fun with food on the weekend, but make sure you follow the *Eating Simply* principles!

FOOD EXERCISE #3

The 85/15 CLUB (or 1 day/week), which graduates to the 92/8 CLUB

Consistency can be the most difficult part of any serious nutritional change. It may be easy to change for 1 day, 1 week, or even 1 month. But as you know, a true lifestyle change is our goal. You may be saying to yourself, " I can't be perfect forever! It's just too hard…"

Well, I don't want you to be perfect forever. I am not so naïve to believe that life doesn't interrupt your health and nutrition goals. If you can eat well in short spurts, great! But what I really want you to shoot for is the 85/15 Club or the 92/8 Club.

SUN MON TUES WED THUR FRI SAT!!!

The numbers refer to the percentage of time that you are eating simply. If you eat simply for 6 out of the 7 days in the week, then you will be eating well 85 percent of the time. The other 15 percent (as mentioned previously) is life! This is drinks with friends from out of town, birthday dinner with your kids, a retirement party with the office, etc. A little wiggle room allows you to live a "normal life" but still stay focused on the task at hand.

After you master the 85/15 Club and you decide to work towards more results, I recommend you move to the 92/8 Club. Obviously this is eating simply 92 percent of the time, or 13 out of every 14 days.

This takes real planning! Knowing that you only have 1 day of "messing up" forces you to really crack down. If you are experienced at eating simply, this can be just a continuation of your normal routine, but if you are new to this, it requires a good amount of discipline.

You will be tempted.

You will be occasionally frustrated.

But you will also realize that once you get into a routine. It is a very rewarding way to live life!

And when life does "happen" and you choose to have a few drinks, or a small slice of that chocolate cake, you will be free of guilt. You no longer need to feel ashamed, guilty, disappointed, or anything else because you know that 92 percent of the time you are feeding your body the nutrition it needs. You are still moving forward and enjoying the fun portions of life!

WARNING: Do not use the 8% or 15% as a constant excuse for not planning ahead, sticking to your goals, and eating the way you can. This is simply a measuring stick so you do not overwhelm yourself and think you can't do this.

• • • TIP Sunday Prep

Spend some time in your kitchen each Sunday to prepare food for the week ahead. Cook 3 or 4 chicken breasts. Create your refrigerator salad bar (see pg.44). Cook some oatmeal. You can reheat what you need in the microwave quickly in the morning. Scramble some eggs and then they are ready to put into a tortilla for a quick breakfast burrito as you head out the door in the morning!

Remember that eating simply takes some planning. If you create the habit of spending just a little time each Sunday to prepare for your week, you will easily achieve the 85/15 club. Habits can be good or bad. Make Sunday prep day a "good habit."

CHAPTER 6

SIMPLY NUTRITIOUS

The pieces to *Eating Simply* are actually very simple. Once you get the hang of this, it becomes very easy to put together simple, nutritious meals for yourself and for your family.

Macronutrients: Carbs, Protein, Fat

There are three main macronutrients: Carbohydrates, Protein, and Fat. Each are digested and used by our body differently, and they are all important to eat. We should never completely eliminate any one of them if we want to support our bodies with the nutrition needed for optimal health.

Carbohydrates: Used for cellular energy among other functions. They are often categorized as simple and complex carbs. Simple carbs have a high glycemic value, rapidly raising your blood sugar, causing you to later crash and feel sluggish. They are converted to fat easier; they do not aid in increasing your metabolism and they commonly have low nutritional value. Examples are white breads and pastas, and sugars like high fructose corn syrup. Complex carbs generally have a lower glycemic value due to higher fiber content, aiding in digestion, allowing you to feel full and energized longer along with being nutrient dense. They are also digested at a higher caloric output, helping you increase your metabolism. Examples are whole wheat products, fruits and veggies, and oatmeal.

Protein: Essential for muscle building and repair. Appropriate amounts help create and maintain lean body mass which supports a higher metabolism in addition to helping stabilize blood sugar.

Consumption is crucial after a workout. Best sources include animal products such as milk, eggs, meat, and fish. Other options include nuts and legumes. The majority of your protein needs to come from lean sources.

Fat: Often criticized, fat is needed just as much as the other two macronutrients. Fat is used for energy storage, insulation, hormone transport and many other things. The 3 commonly mentioned types of fat in our diet are saturated fat, unsaturated fat, and trans fat. Saturated fat is solid at room temperature. Examples include butter and animal fat. Unsaturated fat is liquid at room temperature and should be the higher percentage of your fat intake because of its heart health benefits, such as increasing your HDL (good) cholesterol. Examples include olive oil, plant fats like avocados, and fish oils. Trans fat is man made and is not recognized by your body as food. Therefore, it should NEVER be consumed.

WATER . . . The Fourth Essential Ingredient
This is about as simple as it gets . . . what to drink with lunch? Water. What to drink with dinner? Water. What to have at your desk as you work? Water. You don't need soda. You don't need caffeine if you are eating well, exercising regularly and including appropriate recovery into your routine. Your body needs water for almost every vital function. And even though this may sound counter-intuitive, if you are bloated and holding water for whatever reason, drink more water. It will actually encourage your body to let go of the retained fluid.

I know you have heard that you should drink 8 glasses of water each day. There really is more to it than this, but it is a good common sense place to start. It really depends on your activity level, plus your own body's penchant for releasing water through sweat. The simple idea is . . . drink water instead of soda, or coffee, or tea, or juice, or alcohol, or anything else!

TIP

Is drinking water too boring for you?

Add a slice of lemon to each glass.
Add a slice of orange to each glass.
Add ice cubes.
Use a special glass.
Use a colorful bottle.
Drink through a straw.

I live in Colorado and our water tastes great here. If your water is not so great tasting (and I have experienced this in some of my travels!), invest in a water dispensing machine and get 5 gallon bottles of spring water delivered to your home. Yes, it's more expensive and you will hear lots of arguments that bottled water is no better than tap water . . . but if the bottled water encourages you to drink more because it tastes better, then don't worry about what "everyone else is saying!" Just drink more water.

THE PICK AND CHOOSE LIST OF MACRONUTRIENTS

Pick one ingredient from each list. Grill the meat, steam the vegetables, prepare the starch and add a little fat for flavor. Now that's eating simply!

PROTEIN

Chicken Breast
Turkey
Lean Beef
Buffalo
Tuna
Shrimp
Wild Salmon
Halibut
Eggs
Beans

FIBROUS CARB:

Asparagus	Arugula
Peppers	Kale
Broccoli	Mushrooms
Brussel Sprouts	Tomatoes
Cauliflower	Zucchini
Cabbage	Yellow Squash
Carrots	Spaghetti Squash
Beets	Endive
Celery	Romaine Lettuce
Green Beans	Cucumber
Spinach	

FAT:

Avocado
Olive Oil
Flaxseed Oil
Nuts
Butter
Cream
Cheese

STARCHY CARB:

Brown Rice
Potatoes
Sweet Potatoes
Yams
Oats
Whole Wheat
Quinoa

FOOD EXERCISE #4

"Start with Vegetables" Day

Commonly, when planning our meals at home, my spouse will ask me what I would like to eat on a particular evening. My most common response? I'll say some kind of meat/protein followed by some kind of complex carb. For example, I'll say, "Grilled chicken with bell peppers" or "Salmon and brown rice with a side salad."

You may have gone through a similar scenario, and it's not the wrong way to approach a meal. However, it's good to occasionally challenge your meal thought process by changing the order in which you pick your food.

Your task: plan all of your meals by beginning with veggies. For example, for dinner, choose a medley of cucumbers, carrots, and asparagus. Then determine what proteins and possibly starchy carbohydrates effectively combine with them. BBQ chicken? Lean Steak? Fresh fish? All are good choices, but the centerpiece of your meal is the veggies.

This exercise is difficult! It will take you out of your food comfort zone and force you to try new vegetables.

The purpose of the "Start with Veggies" day is to have you focus on a variety of vegetables, giving your body a wide range of nutrients from different sources. Too often, the powerful complex carbohydrate known as the vegetable can be an after thought. Use this exercise to change that fast!

The Eating Simply Refrigerator Salad Bar

This idea was inspired by my mentor, Phil Kaplan. You can make your own refrigerator into a ready-to-go salad bar. Go to the grocery store and buy all the "goodies" such as:

Lettuce
Spinach
Carrots
Eggs
Cucumbers
Cherry Tomatoes
Red Cabbage
Chicken breast
Avocados
Beets
Mushrooms

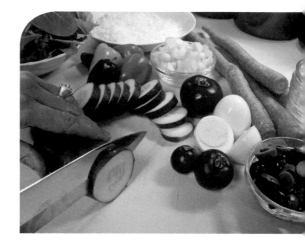

Then prepare all the ingredients. Bake the chicken and cut it into slices. Wash the greens (if necessary). Hard boil the eggs and chop. Chop all the "topping" vegetables. Now put all these ingredients into stackable food containers and stick them into your refrigerator. Your salad bar is ready!

And your mid-day meals are easy to prepare, yummy and supportive of your healthy eating goals.

• • • **TIP** Use the ingredients in your "salad-bar" to make a quick (and simple) omelette/scramble in the morning. Crack a couple eggs in a pan, throw in a couple veggies and a delicious, healthy breakfast is ready in less than 5 minutes.

When you have these ingredients ready ahead of time, breakfast can become simple too. No excuses for not eating well in the morning!

The Eating Simply Stir Fry Dinner

Stir fry for dinner can be really simple and very healthy! It's a lot like the Refrigerator Salad Bar. Make sure you have some of these ingredients available in your refrigerator:

Thin, lean beef strips
Chicken tenderloins
Shrimp
Cabbage or broccoli slaw mix
Bean Sprouts
Green onions
Carrots
Snow peas
Mushrooms
Cashews
Bell peppers of all colors
Soy Sauce
Crystallized ginger
Hoisin Sauce
Pineapple

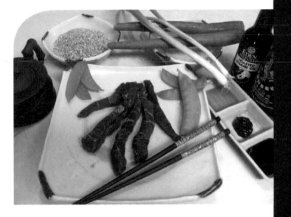

You don't need to have a wok . . . any large skillet will do. The most important thing is to have all of the ingredients that you choose to include in your stir fry meal already cut up before you start cooking.

Chop your meat choice and set it aside in a bowl. Mix a small amount of soy sauce with some corn starch or arrowroot powder. Pour this over the meat and let it marinate while you cut up your vegetables.

Choose 3 or 4 of the vegetables listed. Stir fry is much more interesting with lots of different textures and colors. Chop the vegetables into bite size pieces.

Using a small amount of peanut oil in your skillet, pre-heat the oil for about a minute until it is very hot. Add your vegetables all at once. Stir constantly and cook for just a couple of minutes. Remove the vegetables from the pan and keep warm. Add a little bit more oil to the pan and add the meat with the soy sauce mixture. Cook until done, about 5-6 minutes. Add a little bit of water and some hoisin sauce. Be careful with the sauce – lots of sodium! Add the vegetables back to the skillet and mix together with the meat. Add some chopped crystallized ginger, cashews or pineapple if desired. Serve over cooked brown rice . . . or just enjoy it alone without the added starch!

Each time you make your stir fry, you can choose different combinations and you will have endless meal creations.

SAMPLE MEAL IDEAS

Breakfast ideas:

Breakfast burrito (scrambled eggs, small whole wheat tortilla, real cheese, salsa)
Hard boiled egg, whole wheat toast, fresh fruit
Whole wheat toast, peanut butter, 100% fruit jam
Scrambled eggs with spinach, tomatoes and mushrooms
Ham slice, apple slices and cheese
Shrimp cocktail

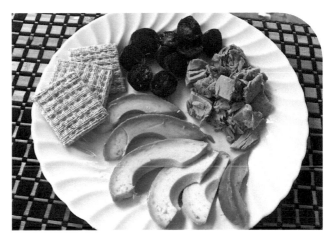

Lunch ideas:
· · · · · · · · · · · · ·

All of the breakfast ideas
Tuna salad, ½ avocado, tomatoes, crackers
Grilled chicken, cubed, with broccoli slaw, dressing
Grilled chicken, pork or beef on a lettuce salad with peas, beets
and tomatoes
Taco salad with ground beef, tomatoes, guacamole, corn, salsa
and a few chips.
Hamburger patty, sweet potato and zucchini
Chicken orzo salad
Spaghetti sauce with ground turkey served over ½ baked potato
Edamame, whole wheat English muffin with peanut butter

Dinner ideas:
· · · · · · · · · · · · ·

All of the breakfast ideas
All of the lunch ideas
Grilled salmon, asparagus and cauliflower
Stir fry with chicken, beef or shrimp and snow peas, broccoli,
carrots, onions and mushrooms. Serve with brown rice.
Turkey soup with rice, tomatoes, onions and zucchini
Whole wheat pasta, grilled chicken, parmesan, asparagus,
and cherry tomatoes.
Steak, lettuce salad and sweet potato

FOOD EXERCISE #5

"Simplify" Your Favorite Food Challenge

Let's face it . . . life without your extra-special favorite lasagna might just be unbearable! But you are realizing that lasagna doesn't exactly fit the "eating simply" mantra. Of course, you can fit your lasagna into the 15% part of your life and "eat simply" the other 85%. But what if it were possible to create a "simple" version of that lasagna that satisfied your craving? It goes like this: Lasagna pans are typically huge. Use a smaller pan so you don't have tons of leftovers and aren't tempted to overeat. Instead of regular lasagna noodles use whole wheat noodles and only do 2 layers instead of three or four. Use one special kind of cheese on the inside and sprinkle the top lightly with parmesan instead of loading up the pan with lots of gooey cheese. And substitute lean ground beef or ground turkey for the fat-laden Italian sausage. And be sure to use canned or boxed tomatoes that are low-sodium instead of the pre-packaged sauce. Now add some fresh herbs to layer with the cheese and the meat sauce. Voila! Simple lasagna that tastes fabulous!

Now you try it for real with one of your favorite dishes. Can you separate a casserole into separate pieces and therefore reduce cooking time and eliminate unnecessary sauces? Or can you reduce the heavy fat and pre-packaged emphasis by changing a recipe like the lasagna example? Try it with just one dish.

I have a favorite chicken recipe from the Crème de Colorado cookbook (*Crème de Colorado* © 1987 Junior League of Denver) that is really not very difficult to begin with, but I simplified it even further. In the original recipe, you have to combine parmesan, bread crumbs, garlic, parsley, oregano, salt and pepper. After dipping the chicken breasts in melted butter, you roll them in the parmesan mixture and then put them in a pan, top with some more butter and bake for 25-30 minutes. Recently, I took some chicken breasts out of the fridge and plopped them into a small casserole dish. I gave them a quick dusting of garlic salt, sprinkled some oregano on top and then some grated pecorino Romano cheese. I poured a small amount of olive oil over the top and baked them for 25-30 minutes. While it was cooking, I cut up some fresh broccoli and steamed it. Dinner was ready in 30 minutes and was really very simple and very nutritious.

The challenge is to find your 3 favorite meals. Tacos, hamburgers, wings, whatever you truly love to eat and push yourself to make it simple. You may find that it really isn't that hard!

It's quite rewarding when you are eating the foods you love, but it is supporting your body, your health, and your metabolism.

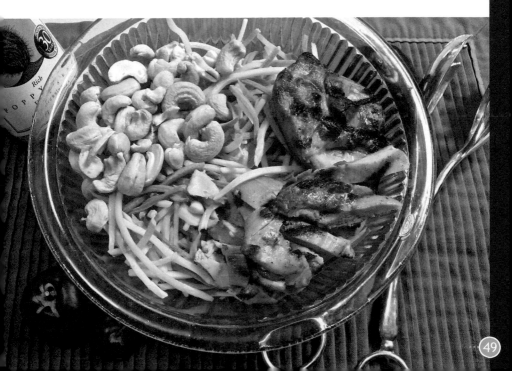

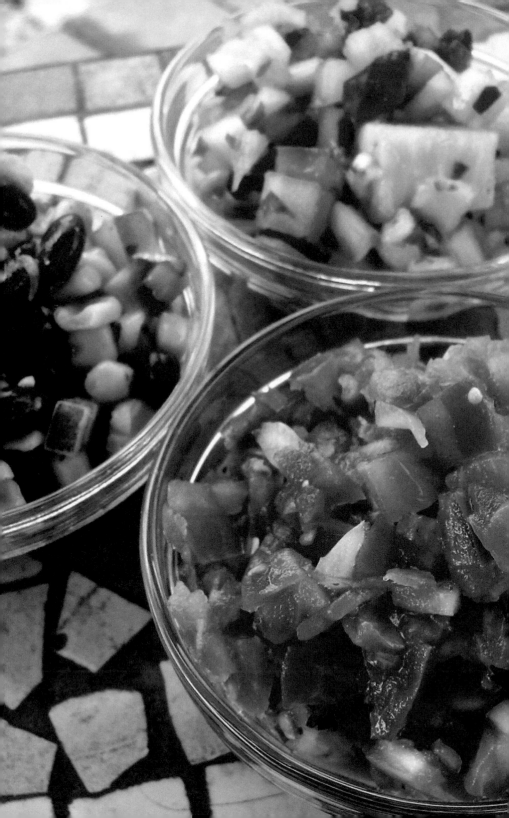

CHAPTER 7

EATING SIMPLY SAUCES

I often hear clients lament, "I'm so tired of plain chicken breast!"
There is no need for you to eat just plain chicken breast . . .
unless you are preparing for a body building show! Spruce up
your chicken – or your fish, turkey, or beef – with these simple to
prepare sauces and salsas. Remember, Eating Simply should be
flavorful!

SALSA ESPECIAL

3 ripe Roma tomatoes
1 small onion
1 tsp chopped garlic
1-2 jalapeño peppers
2 Tbs chopped cilantro
1 small lime
Salt

*Finely chop the tomatoes, onion, garlic and peppers. Mix together
and add the chopped cilantro. Squeeze half a lime over the salsa and
salt to taste.*

MANGO SALSA

2 ripe mangos peeled and cubed
½ cup finely chopped red onion
1 green onion chopped
1 jalapeño finely chopped
Salt

Mix the ingredients in a small bowl. Salt to taste.

TOMATO, OLIVE AND CAPER SAUCE

Inspired from a recipe in *Fine Cooking* Online (*Fine Cooking* ®
Magazine www.finecooking.com).

1 Tbs Olive oil
1 small white onion, diced
2 tsp minced garlic
¾ cup dry white wine
1 tsp dried oregano
½ cup pitted green olives, chopped
1 Tbs capers
15 cherry tomatoes, quartered

*Heat olive oil in skillet over medium heat. Add the onion and cook
until softened, stirring often. Add the garlic and cook about 1 minute. Stir in the wine and oregano, bring to a boil and let cook until
reduced by half. Stir in the tomatoes, olives, and capers and cook for
about 2 minutes. Great with any white fish.*

FRESH TOMATO SAUCE

Prepared tomato sauces are easier and simpler to use for fast
spaghetti sauce. But you have to be careful . . . most of them
contain way more sodium than you need and some of them
actually contain high fructose corn syrup. Here is a simple recipe
for an all-natural tomato sauce that gives you control over the
ingredients.

1 onion, diced
1 Tbs olive oil
7 or 8 medium sized tomatoes, chopped
2 tsp garlic, minced
Fresh basil, oregano and thyme, chopped
Salt to taste

Heat olive oil in skillet over medium heat. Add the onion and cook until softened, stirring often. Add the garlic and cook about 1 minute. Add the chopped tomatoes. Cook for 10 minutes. Add the chopped basil, oregano and thyme and the salt to taste. And for an even easier version . . .
Use canned tomatoes with no sodium added and use dried spices (1 tsp. of each) instead of fresh.

PESTO

These pesto creations can be used to spruce up almost any grilled meat. Or add it to a pasta salad for extra flavor.

2 cups Fresh basil
1/3 cup Pine nuts or walnuts or sunflower seeds
1/3 cup Parmesan cheese or grated Romano cheese
1/3 cup Olive oil
3-4 tsp. garlic
Salt to taste

Add basil and nuts or seeds to a food processor and pulse. Add the garlic and pulse again. Slowly add the olive oil with the food processor on a constant motion. Add the cheese and the salt and combine well.

PEANUT BUTTER AND YOGURT

This is not really a sauce, but rather a dip for fruit slices. Crunchy apples are a great scoop and together this makes a simple, great tasting snack.

½ cup plain Greek yogurt
1/3 cup natural peanut butter

Mix together and serve with apple slices, pear slices, cucumber slices or celery sticks.

PREPARED SALSAS AND SAUCES

Not all prepared items in your grocery store are evil. Salsa is one of the good guys in this arena. You can purchase some really good-for-you salsas. Just take a look at the ingredients and make sure the sodium and sugars are minimal. No high fructose corn syrup!

Barbecue sauce is another great addition, but it can be really difficult to find a sauce that is worthy of the tenets of *Eating Simply*. Learn to read labels and make sure you choose a BBQ sauce that does not include any high fructose corn syrup. You have lots of options here: Kansas City style, St. Louis style, hot, sweet, etc. Your own taste buds will have to guide you here. Add enough for taste . . . but don't overdo it.

• • • **TIP**

Explore the fresh sections in your local grocery store for sauces they prepare right there in the store. Sometimes they will have containers in the produce section. Other times, they will include freshly made sauces next to their meat counter. One other place to look is in the dairy section. If you don't see anything available, ask the grocery manager if they can start including fresh salsas and sauces in their store. Your neighbors will appreciate it as well!

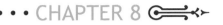

CHAPTER 8

SIMPLY EATING FISH

Want to get more fish oil? Eat Fish!

Don't rely on pills that have processed the fish oil so much its good effects have been minimized. Why not get the oil the way nature intended you to get it . . . by eating fish! Fish is an excellent source of protein and because of our advances in transportation, is readily available even in land-locked areas. And preparing it can be very simple! We asked two local experts to help us understand how to select and then prepare the best tasting fish in our own kitchens.

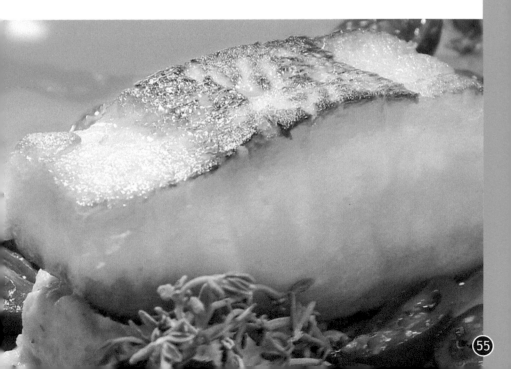

Selecting fresh fish is easy if you know what to look for. Here are some valuable tips:

BUYING WHOLE FISH

Look at the eyes. The eyes should be glossy, bright and clear. Older fish will have eyes with a gray, dull cloudiness and will appear to sink into the carcass. **Next, look at the fish.** Does it shine? Does it look metallic and clean? Never buy fish with dulled skin or has discolored patches on it. **Use the sniff test.** A fresh fish should smell like clean water or even like cucumbers. No pungent aromas! **Look at the gills.** They should be a deep red color. If the fish is old, the gills will turn a dull, purple-brownish color.

BUYING FISH FILLETS

Look for vibrant flesh. If the fillet still has skin, that skin should be shiny and metallic. **Any liquids should be clear.** Liquids on fish should not be milky. Milky liquid on a fillet is the first sign of the fish spoiling.

Buy from a trusted source! If you have a local butcher or seafood market, become friends with them and ask lots of questions. **Local is better!** The farther away it is, the longer it takes to get here. Of course, high end stores fly all their product directly into town within 24-48 hours out of water. **Buy sustainably and wild!** It is our job as consumers to do our part in buying responsibly.

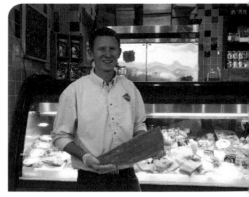

Michael Shepler
Corporate Meat and Seafood Buyer, Tony's Market

Frozen isn't always bad! As a matter of fact, it is sometimes better than fresh. Most frozen-at-sea vessels process and freeze within just a few hours of harvest, preserving the freshness of the fish.

MARCO ISLAND SWORDFISH

IMPORTANT- This one is a bit of extra work- but NOT hard to do! Prep work is very important for this recipe. Make sure all of your ingredients are prepared prior to beginning to cook the fish. It's worth it!

1 lb. Swordfish steaks (or any other white, firm fish like Grouper)
3 slices of bacon
¼ cup finely diced onion
¼ cup finely diced red pepper
¼ cup finely diced mushrooms
¼ cup crab meat (pre-cooked)
1 lb. raw spinach very roughly chopped
1 oz. roughly chunked mozzarella cheese
1 oz. roughly chunked feta cheese
1 tsp butter
Salt

Cook bacon until crisp. Reserve 1 Tbs + 1 tsp of the bacon grease. Crumble/chop the bacon into small crumbles.

Place 1 Tbs of bacon grease in a large skillet and place on medium high heat. Add the swordfish steaks. Cook on each side approximately 4 minutes. Do not overcook.

Place remaining 1 tsp of bacon grease in another large skillet on medium high heat. Heat the onions and red pepper until the onion starts to become transparent. Add the mushrooms and crab meat until heated. Add the spinach and stir until fully wilted. Finally, add the cheese and stir until it starts to melt into the vegetables. Lightly salt and add 1 tsp butter.

Plate the fish and spoon half of vegetable mixture onto the top of the fish. A glass of Pinot Grigio would be a great accompaniment!

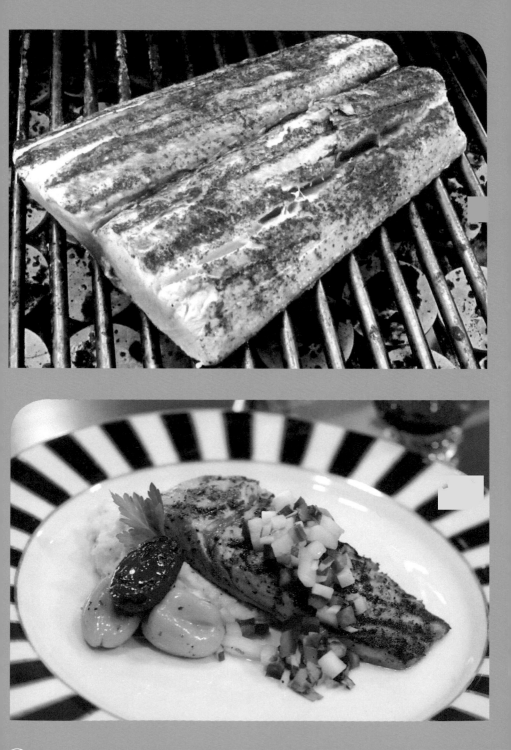

Here are two recipes from Chef Larry DiPasquale.

SALMON AND SONOMA RELISH

Our philosophy has always been pure and simple. Buy wild for the best flavor and sustainability. The bright colors, crisp textures and clean flavors of the relish offset the creamy natural richness of the salmon.

Prepare relish ahead of time by combining all ingredients and refrigerate for 1 hour.

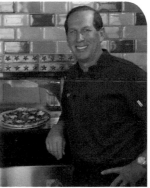

1 cup English cucumber, skin-on, seeded, diced
¾ cup tomato seeded, diced
2 TBL red onion, diced
5 fresh basil leaves, chopped
Juice of one lemon
1 TBL extra virgin olive oil
Balsamic vinegar, to taste
Salt and pepper, to taste

Chef Larry DiPasquale
Owner, Epicurean Catering

4 fresh, wild-caught salmon fillets

The skin helps keep the salmon together on the grill. Check it for pine bones. Remove pine bones with tweezers or clean needle nose pliers. Pat the salmon dry, drizzle it with some extra virgin olive oil and season with sea salt and pepper. Place the salmon on a seasoned grill. To season the grill you can dip a paper towel in oil and, using tongs, rub the oiled towel over the grill. For fillets put the skin side down first. Now don't touch the salmon. The salmon will release itself from the grill when it's ready, usually when it is about 60% done. Using a flat spatula, flip the salmon and cook it to medium rare. For a one inch salmon fillet allow 6 to 10 minutes depending on how done you like it. Once off the grill let it rest a few minutes before serving as it will continue to cook. Plate the salmon and cover with a generous spoonful of the Sonoma Relish. Delish!

SEA BASS WITH TOMATOES AND CAPERS

3 TBL Extra Virgin Olive Oil
4 Black Sea Bass fillets, 6 oz. each, with skin
8 thin lemon slices
8 sprigs fresh Thyme
2 garlic cloves, sliced thin
12 Cherry or Grape tomatoes, halved
1 ½ TBL Capers, drained

Put oven rack in middle position and preheat to 400 degrees. Line a large baking sheet with foil and drizzle with 1 TBL olive oil. Pat fish dry and sprinkle both sides with salt and pepper. Arrange fish, skin down on baking sheet and slide 2 lemon slices under each fillet. Put 2 thyme sprigs on top of each filet.

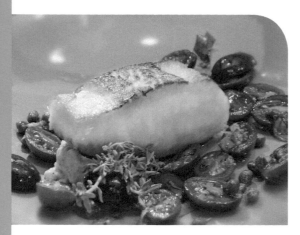

Heat remaining 2 TBL of oil in a 10 inch skillet over medium high heat until it shimmers then sauté garlic until pale golden, about 30 seconds. Add tomatoes and a pinch of salt and sauté 1 minute until tomatoes are soft. Stir in capers.

Spoon hot tomato mixture over fish then cover with another sheet of foil, tenting it and crimping it to form a seal. Bake until fish is just cooked, about 12 to 15 minutes. Check by removing from oven and lifting a corner of the foil to check for doneness. If fish is not done, reseal and check every 3 minutes. Transfer fillets to plates using spatula. Be careful not to tear foil underneath. Spoon tomatoes and juices over fish and serve immediately. Discard thyme before eating.

CHAPTER 9 ⊂═══⬦⊱

RECIPES FOR EATING SIMPLY

Here are some simple go-to recipes that you can start with on your
journey to Eating Simply. You will notice they are not laid out in a
traditional breakfast/lunch/dinner format. You should feel free to
eat any of these recipes at any time of the day you choose. I hope
that as you incorporate these into your life, along with the other
ideas in this book, you will begin to understand that Eating Simply
does not mean boring.

CHICKEN ORZO SALAD

3 boneless, skinless chicken breasts, cooked, chopped
16oz pkg. Dellalo whole wheat orzo
2 carrots, chopped
1 cup canned artichoke hearts, chopped
2 green onions, chopped
1/3 cup kalamata olives, chopped
15 cherry tomatoes, quartered
5-6 TBL. Avocado Vinaigrette (or other Vinaigrette of your choice)

*Cook the orzo
according to the
package. Place
all ingredients
into a large
bowl, add the
dressing to taste
and mix well.
Serve cold.*

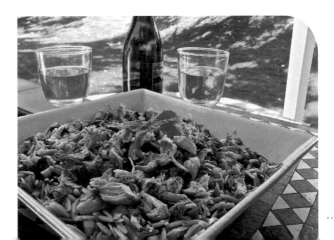

GREEK GRILLED CHICKEN WITH TOMATO-CUCUMBER SALAD

Marinade and Chicken

4 Boneless Skinless Breast Fillets
3 Tbs lemon juice
3 Tbs olive oil
¼ cup chopped flat leaf parsley
1 tsp minced fresh garlic
1 tsp dried oregano
¾ tsp salt
½ tsp ground black pepper

Tomato-Cucumber Salad
1 cup diced fresh plum tomatoes
1 cup diced English cucumber
1 cup diced yellow or red bell pepper
½ cup coarsely chopped pitted Kalamata olives
¼ cup diced red onion
¼ cup crumbled feta cheese

Instructions:
In a medium bowl, combine lemon juice, olive oil, parsley, garlic, oregano, salt and pepper; whisk to blend. Reserve 2 tablespoons marinade for salad. Add chicken to marinade remaining in bowl; turn to coat. Cover and marinate in refrigerator for 30 minutes. Grill chicken over medium heat on outdoor grill or stovetop ridged grill pan for 6 minutes per side or until cooked through.
Meanwhile, in medium bowl combine all tomato-cucumber salad ingredients with reserved 2 tablespoons marinade.
Serve chicken with salad; sprinkle with feta cheese. Garnish with parsley sprigs, if desired. Makes 4 servings.

BAKED OATMEAL

Inspired from a recipe in *Simply Colorado Too!* (© 1999 Colorado Diabetic Association)

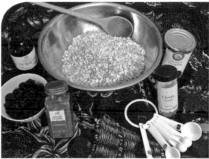

3 cups oats
¼ cup brown sugar
2 teaspoons baking powder
½ teaspoon cinnamon
¼ teaspoon nutmeg
½ teaspoon salt
1 cup milk
½ cup unsweetened applesauce
1 egg + 2 egg whites, lightly beaten
1 teaspoon vanilla extract
1 cup fresh or frozen (thawed) peaches

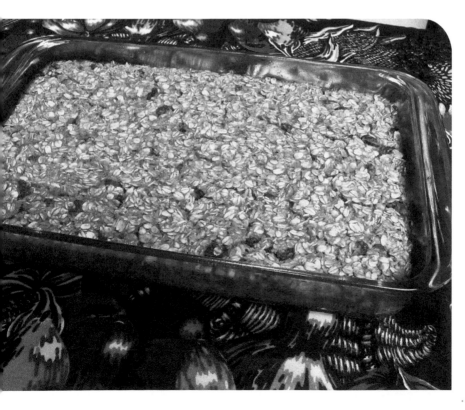

Combine oats, brown sugar, baking powder, cinnamon and salt in a bowl and mix well. Stir in the milk, applesauce, eggs and vanilla. Fold in the peaches. Spread the mixture in a 1 ½ quart baking dish or a 9x9 baking pan sprayed with nonstick cooking spray. Bake at 350 degrees for 30 to 35 minutes.

VARIATION: HARVEST BAKED OATMEAL

4 cups oatmeal
½ cup brown sugar
2 ½ tsp baking powder
1 tsp. pumpkin pie spice
¾ tsp. salt
1 cup milk
1 15oz. can pureed pumpkin (not pumpkin pie mix!)
2 eggs + 2 egg whites
1 tsp. vanilla
½ cup raisins

Combine oats, brown sugar, baking powder, pumpkin pie spice and salt in a bowl and mix well. Stir in the milk, pumpkin, eggs and vanilla. Fold in the raisins. Spread the mixture in a 2 quart baking dish or a 9x13inch baking pan sprayed with nonstick cooking spray. Bake at 350 degrees for 45 minutes.

PROTEIN PANCAKES

4 egg whites
1/3 cup oat bran
⅛ tsp. salt
1 Tbs Honey

Mix everything together and pour into a small, heated skillet that has just a light coating of butter. Cook for about 5 minutes, flip once and finish cooking for another 2-3 minutes. Eat warm with a thin layer of peanut butter or almond butter spread on top!

ROAD WARRIORS

1 cup peanut butter
½ cup honey
1 cup oats, toasted
3 cups oat bran
1 cup protein powder
½ cup coconut milk, unsweetened
Pinch of salt

Mix peanut butter and honey together. Meanwhile toast oats in non-stick pan, stirring constantly until golden brown. Add coconut milk and protein powder to the peanut butter/honey mixture. Add the oats and the pinch of salt. Add the oat bran and mix with your hands. Then turn the mixture out into a 7x12 pan that has been sprayed with oil. Refrigerate for a few hours and then cut into 15 bars.

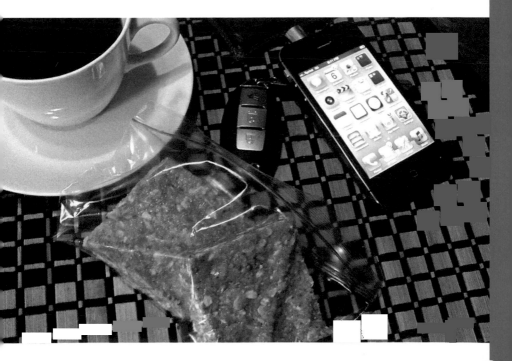

HUMMUS DEVILED EGGS

6 eggs
½ cup hummus
Roasted, salted,
pumpkin seeds

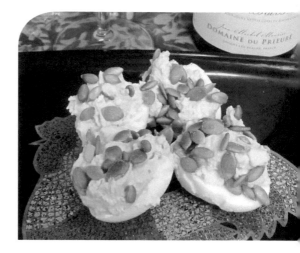

*Boil eggs for 20 minutes.
Drain and cover with
cold water. Lift each egg
out of the cold water after
about 5 minutes and peel.
Cut in half lengthwise
and scoop out the yolk.
Mix the yolks with the hummus and fill each egg-half with some egg
yolk/hummus mixture. Sprinkle pumpkin seeds on top of each egg.*

BROCCOLI SLAW AND CHICKEN

Broccoli slaw (broccoli, carrots, red cabbage)
Roasted chicken, bite sized
Poppy seed dressing
Cashews

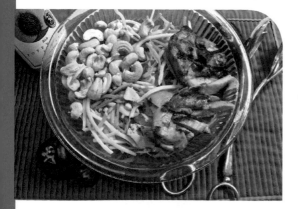

*Combine all ingredients.
Makes an ideal "take to
work" meal. Contains
fibrous carbs, lean protein
and good fats. Needs to be
refrigerated, but not re-
heated to enjoy for a great
supportive, simple meal.*

LENTIL SALAD OVER BAKED POTATO

2 cups cooked brown lentils
½ cup finely diced celery
½ cup finely diced carrot
¼ cup finely diced red onion
½ cup chopped, fresh cherry tomatoes
½ cup canned artichoke hearts, chopped
Chopped, fresh parsley
¼ cup olive oil
2 Tbs lemon juice
2 tsp. minced garlic
¼ tsp. dried thyme
¼ tsp. ground cumin
¼ tsp. salt
Dollop plain yogurt

Combine the cooked lentils with the celery, carrots, onion, tomatoes, artichoke hearts and parsley. In a separate bowl, mix the olive oil, lemon juice, garlic, thyme, cumin and salt and blend vigorously. Pour the olive oil mixture over the lentil/vegetable mixture. Serve over small, baked potatoes with a dollop of plain yogurt on top.

PASTA PIE (A GREAT USE FOR LEFTOVERS!)

½ pound, cooked, whole wheat pasta (linguine, fettuccine, spaghetti, angel hair)
1 egg, 2 egg whites
1/3 cup parmesan cheese
½ cup roasted red bell pepper
1 cup cooked broccoli
¼ cup minced, fresh basil
3 green onions, chopped
2 cups, cooked chicken
½ cup parmesan cheese
½ cup milk
1 egg

Mix the cooked pasta, 1 egg , 2 egg whites and ⅓ cup cheese together and pour into a well-greased 9 inch deep pie plate to form a crust. Mix together the vegetables and chicken. Pour into the prepared pasta crust. Mix ½ cup cheese, milk and egg together and pour over the pie. Cover with greased foil. Bake at 350 degrees for 30 minutes. Remove and let stand for 5 minutes before cutting into pie slices for a yummy dinner!

EDAMAME AND PEANUT BUTTER ENGLISH MUFFIN

An easy, complete snack for work or home! Protein, complex carbohydrate and quality fat!

1 whole wheat English muffin
2 Tbs Natural peanut butter
½ cup frozen edamame

Cook edamame according to package. Toast the English muffin and spread with peanut butter. Spread edamame on top of split English muffin halves and enjoy!

QUICK BLACK BEAN SOUP

1 can no-sodium added black beans
½ cup tomato salsa
1 cup low-sodium chicken broth
1 cup fresh spinach
1 cup cooked chicken
Salt to taste
¼ cup grated jack cheese, optional

Mix all the ingredients together in a sauce pan and heat. Enjoy a quick, healthy lunch or dinner!

EASY CROCK POT GREEN CHILI

3-5 lb. pork shoulder
Chicken broth
28 oz. canned no-sodium added diced tomatoes
10-12 roasted Anaheim chilies
2 tsp salt

Place pork shoulder in a crockpot and cover with chicken broth. Cook on low for 8 hours. Remove pork and reserve broth. Shred pork. Skim fat off of broth.

Peel and chop Anaheim chilies. Place shredded pork, de-fatted broth, tomatoes, salt and chilies into a dutch oven and cook for 30 minutes on the stove-top. Serve with whole wheat tortillas.

BREAKFAST BURRITOS

Easy to make ahead and take with you on the way to school or work!

Whole wheat tortillas
Eggs
Cheese, grated
Ground turkey
Italian seasoning
Salt

Scramble eggs; cook in pan with a small amount of butter and lightly season with salt. Cook ground turkey by sautéing in a skillet and skim off excess fat. Add Italian seasoning.
To assemble burritos, scoop ½ cup scrambled eggs, ½ cup cooked, seasoned, ground turkey and ¼ cup grated cheese on one small, whole wheat tortilla. Fold burrito style. Roll into wax paper. Heat in a microwave oven for 1 minute prior to serving. Freeze remaining burritos.

GRILLED CHICKEN HUMMUS PIZZA

1 whole wheat ready- made pizza dough
Corn meal
Roasted garlic in oil
Sun-dried tomatoes in oil
Ready-made hummus
Roasted chicken
Fresh basil leaves, julienned
Fresh spinach leaves, julienned
Italian spices
Grated parmesan or pecorino Romano cheese

Roll out the pizza dough and sprinkle with corn meal. Pre-heat a gas grill to MEDIUM and place the dough directly on the rack which has been oiled or sprayed with grill oil. Grill for a few minutes until the bottom of the crust is starting to brown. Remove the pizza dough and place on a plate cooked side up. Spread hummus evenly over the dough. Add garlic cloves, sun-dried tomatoes, chicken, basil leaves and spinach leaves. Sprinkle spices liberally over entire pizza. Top with enough cheese to cover lightly. Place pizza back onto the grill and cook for 5-10 minutes until crust is crispy and cheese is melted. Remove from grill, cut into slices and serve immediately.

SCRAMBLED EGGS WITH VEGETABLES

Use your creativity and add any leftover cooked vegetables available in your refrigerator.

1 whole egg
2 egg whites
1 Tbs Olive oil
Vegetables (spinach, mushrooms, broccoli, cauliflower, squash, etc.)
1 oz Chèvre goat cheese
Chopped cherry tomatoes

Heat olive oil in a small skillet. Add ¾ to 1 cup of cooked vegetables and heat thoroughly. Scramble whole egg and egg whites together and add to skillet with cheese. Cook for a couple of minutes until just slightly dry. Serve with chopped tomatoes on top.

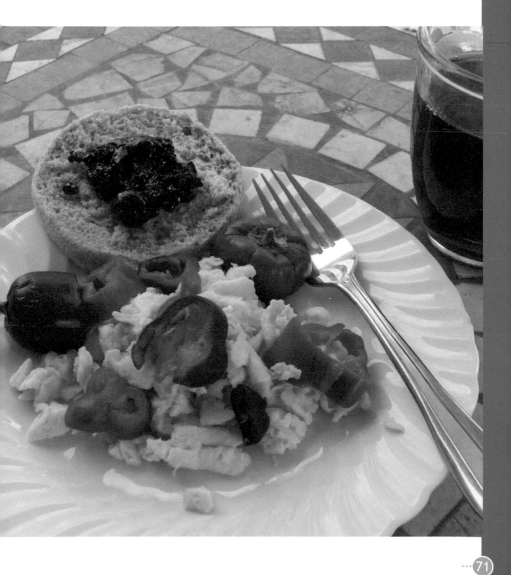

MEXICAN SKILLET DINNER

A great use for leftover roast beef or roasted chicken!
Re-configure and create new tastes for your family!

3 small Zucchini, sliced
1 Tbs Olive oil
1 cup Cooked Black beans (canned or boxed)
½ cup Tomato Salsa or fresh cherry tomatoes, chopped
½ cup Corn (frozen or fresh)
2 cups Roasted chicken or roast beef
1 cup Roasted, chopped Anaheim chili peppers
¼ cup each, Fresh oregano and cilantro, chopped
¾ cup Grated cheese
Whole wheat tortillas or brown rice

*In a large skillet, heat the olive oil and add the sliced zucchini.
Cook for 10 minutes until softened. Add beans, salsa or tomatoes,
corn, chicken or beef, chili peppers, oregano and cilantro. Cook
thoroughly for 5 minutes. Serve with tortillas or on top of cooked
rice and sprinkle with grated cheese.*

CHICKEN AND CAPERS

2 boneless/skinless chicken breasts
¼ cup whole wheat flour
Salt/pepper
Olive Oil
1 Tbs capers
1 tsp lemon juice
1 Tbs whole wheat flour
½ cup chicken stock
Thinly sliced lemon

Heat the skillet on medium high. While your skillet is heating, salt and pepper the chicken breast dredge through the flour. Add the olive oil to skillet and gently sauté the chicken until browned and done through.

Remove the chicken onto a plate and cover to keep warm.
Turn the heat down on your skillet to medium. Add 1 Tbs of flour to the oil in the skillet and stir. Add the chicken stock slowly, stirring as added until it incorporates the flour. Add the capers and lemon juice.

Place a chicken breast on each plate. Spoon the caper sauce over the chicken. Place a lemon slice on the breast.

Serve with brown rice and steamed broccoli.

SUPER EASY CHICKEN AND RICE SOUP

2 chicken breasts, cut into bite sized pieces (Leftover turkey works too!)
4 cups reduced fat/salt chicken broth
½ cup short grain brown rice
1 small onion diced
2 carrots, sliced
1 small zucchini, cubed
Handful of fresh spinach roughly chopped
4-5 cherry tomatoes/ halved.

Bring the broth to a low boil and add the rice, onion and sliced carrots. Allow to simmer for 30 minutes. Add the chicken pieces and zucchini to the broth and simmer for 10 minutes more.

Now add the chopped spinach. Simmer until the spinach is wilted, about a minute.

Finally add the halved tomatoes and serve immediately.

EXPRESS CONGEE

Traditionally a breakfast in the Chinese culture, but can be enjoyed anytime!

Brown rice hot cereal
Chicken broth
Pre-cooked chicken (rotisserie chicken from the market is great!)
Chopped vegetables (green onions, spinach, peppers etc.)
Eggs

Prepare the hot rice cereal as directed.

Put ½ cup of the hot cereal in a microwave safe bowl
Add ¼ cup of chicken broth, a few pieces of cut up, pre-cooked chicken and some of the vegetables.
Cover and heat for a minute in the microwave

Fry, or poach, an egg to medium. Add the egg to the top of the congee and enjoy!

"ITALIAN" CONGEE

Ok, a bit of "license" here, but you will enjoy this tremendously for its flavor and ease of preparation!

3 cups water
1 cup polenta (corn grits)
1 Tbs butter
½ tsp salt

Bring the water to a boil in a medium saucepan. Add the polenta and salt slowly while constantly whisking to prevent clumping. When all of the polenta is incorporated, add the butter and stir. Cover and let sit until the shrimp is ready.

12 large shrimp
1 Tbs. butter
1 cup dry white wine
Salt
Fresh herbs (dill, tarragon, parsley, basil, rosemary - whatever you have on hand) (Reserve a tablespoon or so for garnish)

Sauté the shrimp in butter until pink. Add the wine and salt and bring to a boil. Add the herbs, cover and simmer for a minute or two.

Place about ½ cup of the polenta in a bowl. Add 3 shrimp and a good portion of the "sauce" left in the skillet. Sprinkle with fresh herbs and serve hot.

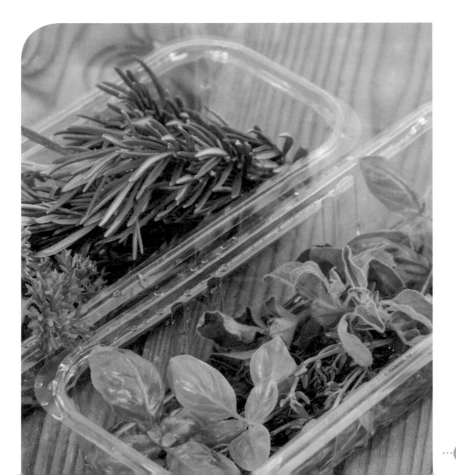

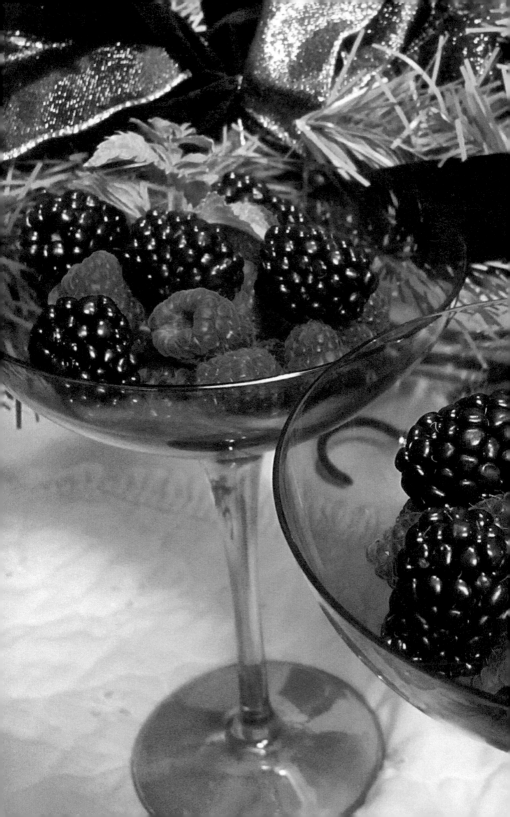

CHAPTER 10

SIMPLY SWEET

Let's face it, sometimes you just need something sweet. Not a lot, I know. But it just "finishes" the palate nicely. Here are a few ideas for sweet treats that really are very simple!

Eating Simply with a Sweet Tooth

Fresh berries with a little cream (real cream . . . not that fake stuff)
Crystallized ginger chunks
Watermelon
Peaches
Plums
Pears
Pineapple
Grapes
All of the above mixed into a fruit salad
Dates
Orange slices
Mint tea w/sugar

And for the adults . . .
A cup of coffee with a splash of Kahlua or Bailey's
A dessert wine
A glass of port or cognac

And finally, here are a few simple recipes for desserts:

MANGO "ICE CREAM"

10 oz frozen mango chunks
1/3 cup sugar
1 cup coconut milk
1 tsp lemon juice
½ tsp kosher salt

Put frozen mango chunks in the bowl of a food processor. Pulse until well chopped. Add sugar, lemon juice and salt. Pulse until blended.

Turn on processor and add Coconut milk in a steady stream until blended and smooth.

Transfer to a bowl and place in the freezer for about ½ hour.

Stir, then serve.

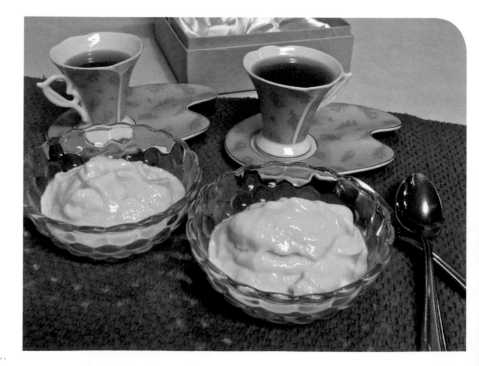

STRAWBERRY SHORTCAKE

Instead of using a true shortcake which is laden with butter, substitute lighter Angel Food cake.

Fresh or frozen strawberries
Angel food cake
Real Whipped cream

If your strawberries are fresh, wash them thoroughly and then trim the stem off and cut into sections. If you add just a small dusting of sugar to the berries, they will "sweat" and create a nice sauce effect for the dessert. Cut small sections of Angel food cake and cover each slice with a generous helping of strawberries. If desired, add a small amount of whipped cream on top for an elegant, easy dessert.

BAKED APPLES

This one takes some time to cook, but is easy to prepare and full of comfort for Fall!

4 baking apples (Granny Smith, Rome, etc)
¼ cup brown sugar
1 tsp cinnamon
¼ cup chopped nuts (pecans, walnuts etc)
⅓ cup raisins or dried cranberries (or mixed)
4- thin slices of butter (about ¼" thick each)
1 cup boiling water

Leaving the peel on the apple, core removing about ¾ in hole down the middle of the apple.

Mix all of the remaining ingredients except the butter and boiling water. Stuff each apple with this mixture.

Place a slice of butter on the top of each apple's stuffing.

Put the stuffed apples in a shallow baking dish that is large enough to hold all the apples. Pour the boiling water beside the apples, and place the baking dish in a 375 degree oven for 40 minutes. Serve warm.

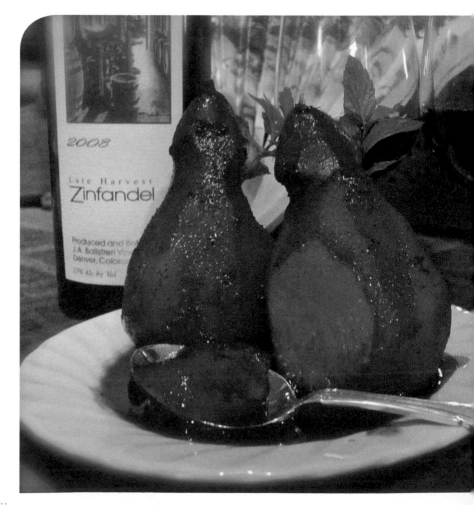

POACHED PEARS

4 pears (Bosc or Anjou)
1 ½ cups of red wine (a sweeter zinfandel will work here or better yet, a port)
½ cup sugar
Juice of ½ lemon + 1 tsp of zest
1 tsp cinnamon
½ tsp ground cloves
1 tsp vanilla

Leaving the stem intact, peel the pears and slice a small piece off the bottom (so it can sit up straight). Set aside.

Put the next 5 ingredients in a sauce pan that is just big enough around to hold the pears standing up. Bring to a boil then simmer for a few minutes.

Stand the pears in the simmering sauce, cover the pan and allow to cook for 20-25 minutes (until soft but not mushy) Remove the pears to individual bowls.

Bring the remaining sauce to a boil and reduce until ⅓ volume remains.

Pour the sauce over the pears.

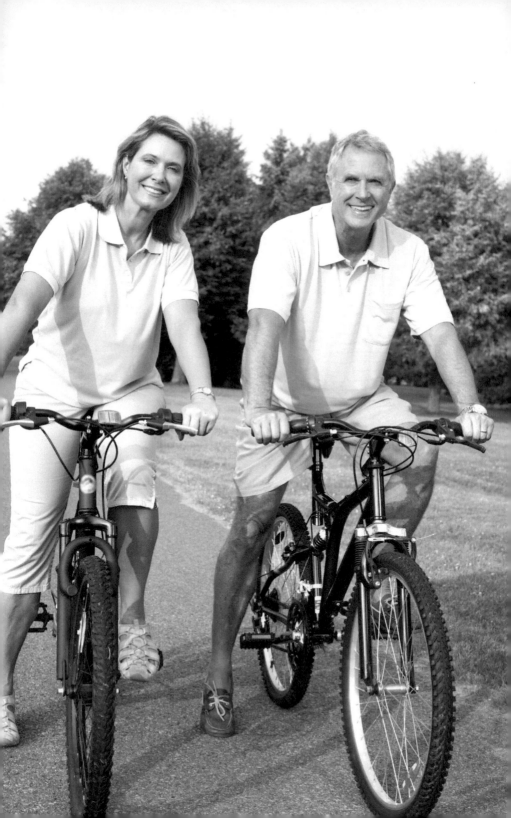

LIVING SIMPLY

No, I'm not going to get on my soapbox and ask you to go live in a commune somewhere . . . but that just shows that I lived in the 1960's, doesn't it? Living simply is an idea that can be fleshed out in your own way. When you can end each day with a contented sigh and be fully convinced that it was a good day . . . you have mastered the art of living simply.

Eating Simply in your 20's, 30's, 40's and beyond

Grant:
Being in my 20's, I understand that I can "get away" with eating poorly. I can choose to eat like the majority of my peers and worry about the consequences later. However, I choose to eat simply to build a foundation for later in life. I understand the choices I make today affect me later. Don't read this wrong: I make mistakes and I am not perfect, but my wife and I continually try to eat better each and every week. We work on our "nutritional balance," allowing us to enjoy the fun side of youth. The 85/15 club is a great tool for us. But I constantly challenge myself to find delicious, simple foods and meals that will help improve our lives. We choose to eat simply for our health, our vitality and for our future.

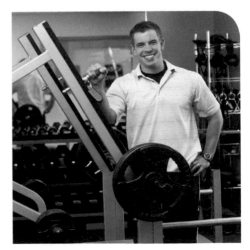

Dianne:

Since I have successfully completed 5 decades of life, I can give you a "20/20 hindsight" look at eating through the years. I remember in my 20's not really caring what I ate. Food needed to taste good, and it needed to be convenient, but those really were the only criteria. Well, I guess food also needed to be affordable! But I certainly didn't see the connection between how my body looked

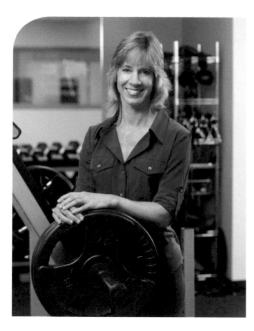

and what I was feeding it. I didn't connect energy levels or mental acuity with what I was putting into my body. Certainly, I started to think about nutrition when my kids came along. I wanted to make sure I was giving them the best start possible. But it didn't really click with me until I was in my 40's, when my exercise and my nutrition combined, and my body started to respond. I looked and felt better than when I was in my 20's. You may not see or feel the effects of what you are eating when you are in your 20's, but believe me, every time you choose fast food, you are wreaking havoc on your body. If I could say one thing only, it would be to pay attention to your body and eat well from the beginning. The sooner you adopt these *Eating Simply* principles, the better your body will be able to handle stress, pregnancy, illness, and anything else life throws at you.

YOUR NEXT STEP:
. . . .

You have choices every day. Commit now to Eating Simply and you will be amazed at how this affects the rest of your life. Eat better this week than you did last week. Continue forward, always trying to improve your nutrition. You will handle the stress of each new endeavor with energy, resilience and strength. And aging will become a game . . . with twists and turns certainly, but fun all the same!

So get started today and begin eating simply!

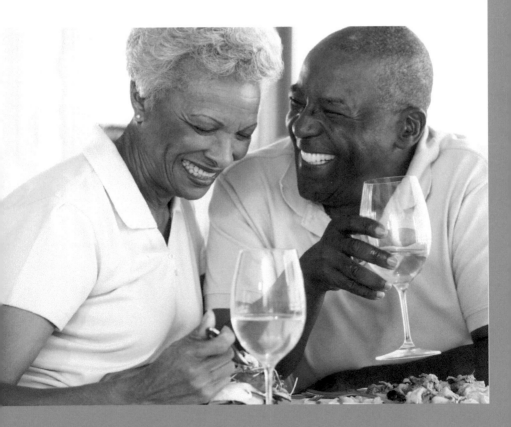

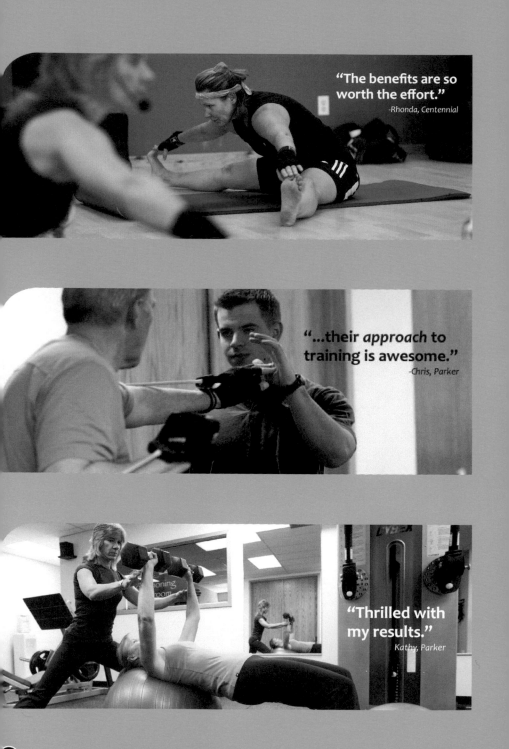

"The benefits are so worth the effort."
-Rhonda, Centennial

"...their *approach* to training is awesome."
-Chris, Parker

"Thrilled with my results."
Kathy, Parker

AFTERWORD

EXERCISING SIMPLY

Embracing the concepts of *Eating Simply* will help you create a healthy body now and will guard that health through the years to come. However, it would be irresponsible if we didn't mention that exercising also has to be a regular part of your life. Looking and feeling your best becomes easy when you balance the right nutrition and the right exercise.

Exercising Simply will become a book on its own. However, we wanted to give you a few tips to help you evaluate your current program and begin to get on the right track.

Here are the 4 things every exercise program needs:

Aerobic exercise - Include both steady-state exercise and interval training to build and strengthen your cardiovascular system.

Resistance Training - Challenge the muscles to spur positive growth in strength, functionality, and metabolism.

Flexibility Training - To maintain functional range of motion, allowing you to do the things you love.

Proper Recovery - Without rest, the body can't "process" the workout. Results come from recovery.

Effectively combine all 4 to ensure a balanced and complete program.

So take a second and think about your current exercise program. Do you incorporate all 4 factors? Are you missing 1 or 2? Or maybe you're not exercising at all?

We'll discuss each of these components in depth in our next book, *Exercising Simply*. We want to take the advertising hype and mystery out of moving your body effectively so you can achieve that vibrant, full life you have been dreaming about.

Contact a professional personal trainer in your area to help you understand and implement the concepts of *Exercising Simply*. You simply can't continue to exercise like you did in high school and expect the results that you want as an adult.

If you can't wait for *Exercising Simply* and have questions regarding eating or exercising simply, give us a call at 303-522-9001 or visit www.theconditioningclassroom.com.

If you live in the Denver area, you can claim a free, 30-minute consultation to visit The Conditioning Classroom and ask us your exercise questions face-to-face. Call 303-522-9001 to schedule an appointment or sign up online at www.theconditioningclassroom.com.

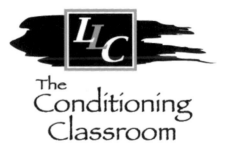

The
Conditioning
Classroom

www.theconditioningclassroom.com

Do you have a group that would benefit from learning how to eat and exercise simply?

You can have Dianne or Grant teach the principles of living simply at your next event.

If you would like Dianne or Grant to speak to your group or conference please send an email with details on the date, the group etc to:

grantp@theconditioningclassroom.com

or

dbailey@theconditioningclassroom.com

••• **TIP**

And if you have enjoyed the ideas and recipes of *Eating Simply*, sign up for our newsletter at www.theconditioningclassroom.com to receive new ideas twice a month.

Help spread the idea that living well can be simple!

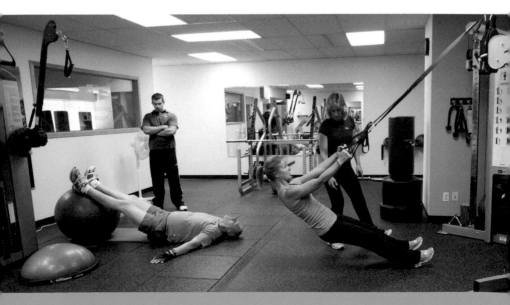

DIANNE BAILEY, CSCS

Dianne has been providing professional weight management and sports conditioning training for individuals since 2002 and opened The Conditioning Classroom in 2006. Her personal journey into the world of fitness began in 1994 when she took her first self-defense class in Gracie Jiu-jitsu. She was hooked and has stayed active in the martial arts, earning her 4th degree black belt in Taekwondo in 2008. Along the way, she has taken classes in Krav Maga, Hapkido, Tai Chi, American Boxing and is currently Denver's premiere kickboxing instructor, having taught classes since 1998. She has been featured in and contributed articles to the Denver Post and the Examiner, has been a guest on 9News, has produced 2 exercise DVD's (Every Day Flexibility and COREiculum) and is the author of a 12-week exercise and nutrition program called The Revolution.

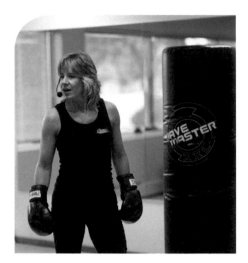

Dianne is also a participant in a national coalition of 10-12 elite personal trainers called the Be Better Platinum project headed by renowned trainer Phil Kaplan. This group interacts regularly to push each other in a quest to raise the bar of professionalism for the personal training industry and to create a level of public awareness that personal trainers are an integral component of health care.

She has recently been asked to become a member of the advisory committee for Arapahoe Community College's Human Performance/ Exercise Health Sciences department.

She lives in Denver with her husband, Jim, and her business partner is her younger son, Grant. Her older son, Ben, lives in Seattle and works in the aerospace industry.

GRANT PETTEGREW, CSCS

Grant has been helping people exercise/eat the correct (and simple) way, allowing them to look and feel their best since 2008. Grant graduated from Colorado State University with a degree in health and exercise science, and is an NSCA Certified Strength and Conditioning Specialist.

Grant is also an avid golfer whose passion for fitness has helped him and many others enjoy the game more. His education has allowed him to understand the golf swing and the physical demands it brings. He is devoted to teaching golfers how to take control of their bodies and their

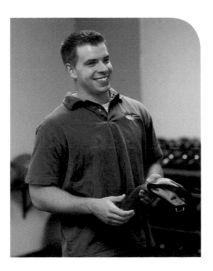

game. Grant has had articles published in multiple golf magazines, including Colorado Avid Golfer, and has been featured on Denver's 9News for golf fitness.

That love of golf and fitness has continued today, leading him to create www.golfconditioningnow. com and author 2 "on your own" workout guides for golfers: *The Total Golf Workout* and *The Beginner Golf Workout*.

Grant lives in Parker with his wife, Andrea and their dog, Max (who has his own column in Golf Conditioning Now's monthly newsletter.) Each week they plan their meals out ahead of time, helping each other stay accountable to the principles of *Eating Simply*.

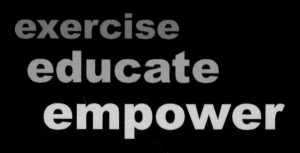

exercise
educate
empower

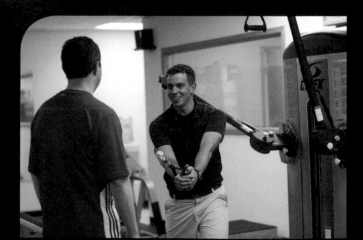

"The only Nutrition book you'll ever need! This book sums up the specifics of how to eat healthy, and clears up all the misconceptions surrounding food. Loaded with truth and real world application, this book is one of my favorites in a long time. EVERYONE should own this book, it's right on!"

- Jim Beatty, CSCS, CPT
Owner, FitnWell
Philadelphia, PA

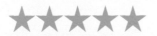

"Dianne and Grant summarize the principles of Eating Simply so... well, simply! With all the diet books, programs, and companies hyping their particular "solution" to our weight problems, eating disorders, and nutritional challenges, Dianne and Grant unravel a complex subject into very manageable, uncomplicated chunks of digestible information.

I particularly enjoy the simple sauce recipes. Eating simply clearly does not mean boring!"

- David N. Kwiecinski
Personal Trainer, Health and Fitness Consultant
Chicago, IL

"This book is filled with so much useful information about how to eat better (including loads of easy and healthy recipes); plus, it is extremely easy (and fun!) to read: it's written very clearly, and they also did a great job of formatting the information into bite-size pieces. The colors, graphics, and overall format of the book make it so fun to work with. I read the book cover-to-cover, and I keep it in my kitchen as a daily go-to guide for reference and inspiration."

- Dr. Sarah Pessin
Denver, CO

"I really appreciate this book. It is an easy "go to" for meal ideas that use healthy "real" food without too any ingredients or ingredients you normally wouldn't have on hand. Some of these recipes are now on my weekly list and make me feel good about what I feed my family."

- Linda Harrison
Occupational Therapist
Englewood, CO